ACUPUNCTURE
FOR AMERICANS

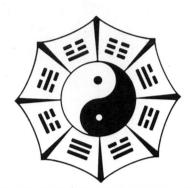

ACUPUNCTURE FOR AMERICANS

Louise Oftedal Wensel, M.D.

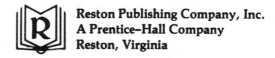

Reston Publishing Company, Inc.
A Prentice–Hall Company
Reston, Virginia

Library of Congress Cataloging in Publication Data

Wensel, Louise O
   Acupuncture for Americans.

   Includes index.
   1. Acupuncture.   I. Title.   [DNLM:
1. Acupuncture.   WB369 W476ab]
RM184.W443   615.8'92   80-12800
ISBN 0-8359-0127-0

© 1980
Reston Publishing Company, Inc.
A Prentice–Hall Company
Reston, Virginia 22090

10   9   8   7   6   5   4   3   2   1

Printed in the United States of America

CONTENTS

PREFACE

This book is an attempt to integrate the practice of acupuncture with American medical science. It can be used to teach acupuncture to physicians, medical students, nurses, and medical technicians.

Since its language is as free from medical jargon as possible, the author hopes that most of it will be understandable to Americans who do not have special medical training. It should enable them to determine whether acupuncture is likely to be a safe and effective treatment for their specific medical problems.

Some people may even be able to use this book to learn how to give themselves, or their relatives and friends, temporary relief from pain by giving acupressure at some of the points listed for treating certain painful conditions.

Before prescribing dangerous drugs or surgery, physicians should be sure that a safer treatment, such as acupuncture, would not be at least as effective for treating a patient's ailment. Physicians have an obligation to continue their medical educations and to acquire knowledge about every treatment which might benefit their patients. Those who use their ignorance of acupuncture as an excuse for condemning it, or not recommending it for appropriate cases, are negligent and too closed-minded to be considered scientific.

Acupuncture is not a panacea or cure-all. It is simply a modality of safe, inexpensive medical treatment which can be effective in many situations, sometimes in combination with other treatment. It can become readily available and no longer seem mysterious if it is taught to American medical personnel. The limitations of acupuncture and precautions about its use described in this book, however, should be given careful consideration.

One of the reasons that American medical scientists give for ignoring the possibilities of acupuncture is that no textbook meeting the standards of American medical science is available in English. Too many books on acupuncture are mainly translations of Oriental texts which include philosophy, religion, or political propaganda mixed with science. Others are anecdotal and give little useful information.

I am very grateful to my American medical colleagues who have shown an interest in acupuncture and given me valuable suggestions and criticisms in preparing this book. They have kept me mindful of the advanced state of American medical technology and of the excellent drugs for treating specific diseases.

Many Chinese translators and acupuncturists have helped me assemble the information about acupuncture. I have enjoyed working with them and developed great respect for their culture and their ability to adapt to American culture.

The ancient Chinese treatises on acupuncture are in classical Chinese, which has more elaborate characters and is more abstruse than that used after Yat-sen Sun, M.D., attempted to modernize the language when he was president of China in the 1920's. Chinese characters have been further simplified since Mao's "Cultural Revolution" and are now written across a page like English instead of in vertical columns as previously. Since the Chinese language does not have an alphabet, it is difficult to look up Chinese words in a dictionary.

Difficulty in translating from Chinese is probably one of the reasons Americans have tended to ignore Chinese medical literature. Now that the Chinese have officially adopted the Pinyin system of Romanizing a standard spoken language, thus replacing their many regional dialects, communication with the Chinese may be facilitated.

Besides adding the Chinese medical art of acupuncture to our medical armamentarium, I wish we would add the Chinese word *ta* to our English vocabulary. This little word means "he, him, she, her, or it." Since English does not have a single pronoun which can be used to refer to a *person*, male or female, I have to state that all male pronouns used in this book should be considered female as well.

PART 1

A COMPREHENSIVE INTRODUCTION TO ACUPUNCTURE

chapter 1

ACUPUNCTURE
IN AMERICA

The Chinese medical art of inserting fine needles into the skin to relieve pain or disability was practiced in the United States more than 150 years ago. In 1826 the *North American Medical and Surgical Journal* published an article entitled, "Cases Illustrative of the Remedial Effects of Acupuncture."[1] Many Chinese immigrants brought their acupuncture needles with them when they came here in the nineteenth century but used them mostly on their families and friends. At the turn of the century, however, Dr. William Osler of Johns Hopkins Medical School recommended it in his medical textbooks.[2]

Television and other publicity resulting from former president Richard M. Nixon's 1972 trip to China introduced millions of Americans to the possibilities of acupuncture. A few months later the first acupuncture center opened in Washington, D.C., followed by the establishment of acupuncture centers in many other localities. Many Americans have already obtained lasting relief from their pains and disabilities through acupuncture. Some American physicians have used acupuncture analgesia successfully for childbirth, including Caesarean sections, and for other surgical procedures.

A few medical schools now offer courses in acupuncture. Various medical organizations have offered symposia on acupuncture to physicians for continuing medical education credit. Some Americans have traveled to Oriental or European countries for courses in acupuncture.

The use of transcutaneous electric stimulation (TES) at acupuncture points, electro-acupuncture, has been shown to cause the brain and other organs to produce morphine-like biochemicals.[3] As research on these biochemicals (endorphins and enkephalins) continues, increasing numbers of medical scientists are becoming interested in acupuncture for relief of depression and mental illness as well as pain.[4] This research is discussed further in Chapters 5 and 9.

Chiropractors have developed techniques for "acupressure" to circumvent legal prohibitions against their piercing the skin. They have also used the probes of electric point-finding instruments to give "electro-acupressure." Some patients have learned to give themselves acupressure for temporary pain relief.[5] TES equipment does not necessarily pierce the skin.

MEDICAL NEEDS WHICH CAN BE MET BY ACUPUNCTURE

In spite of the excellence of American medical technology and pharmacology, there are still some important medical needs which can be met by acupuncture. These include (1) analgesia for surgery and chronic pain syndromes which is safe as well as effective, (2) somatic psychiatric treatment which does not cause brain damage, allergies, or other undesirable side effects, (3) therapy to relieve the symptoms of neurologic disorders which have been labeled hopeless, and (4) effective treatment for chronic allergies without the hazards of desensitizing injections or drugs.

The chemicals American physicians use for analgesia are toxic. Most of the operating room deaths in the United States are caused by anesthesia rather than by surgery.[6] Narcotic, hypnotic, and tranquilizing drugs produce many side effects as well as addiction. The most effective drugs for treating arthritis can cause symptoms more serious than the disease and can sometimes cause fatal illness. There are no drugs which are effective for treating many disabling neurologic disorders. Some allergic patients have anaphylactic reactions to desensitizing injections. They may become too drowsy to drive or work if they take antihistamines.

Acupuncture can be useful for coping with all of these medical problems if it is practiced in accordance with American standards of asepsis by well-trained acupuncturists. It does not produce allergic reactions or other undesirable side effects. Although acupuncture may give adequate analgesia for major surgery if the patient is co-operative and the acupuncturist is skillful enough, it cannot produce unconsciousness. It is less dependable than anesthetic drugs or narcotics for temporary relief of surgical or other severe pain but may reduce the quantity of these drugs required.

LIMITATIONS OF ACUPUNCTURE

There are many medical conditions for which acupuncture should not be used in the United States, although early Chinese textbooks indicate that this treatment modality was regarded as a complete system of medical practice. Even in China, however, it has been supplemented for hundreds of years with herbology. More recently, it has been supplemented by drugs and modern surgical techniques. Acupuncture is mainly useful for analgesia and treating chronic conditions which have been thoroughly diagnosed by American physicians.

Chinese pulse diagnosis is of doubtful validity as well as being extremely difficult to learn. Although it has been closely associated with acupuncture and traditional acupuncturists consider it essential before each treatment, it should certainly not replace more precise and extensive American diagnostic techniques.

Another Chinese technique traditionally associated with acupuncture is moxibustion, the burning of the herb *Artemesia vulgaris* (*Moxa*) over the acupuncture site. The marijuana-like aroma and the heat are thought to potentiate the effects of acupuncture. The hazards of moxibustion, however, make it inappropriate for American use.

In general, acupuncture should not be used to treat any condition in the United States for which there is already a safe and effective treatment available. It should not be used to treat any type of tumor or to delay getting diagnostic studies and standard American treatment for any symptom which might be an indication of cancer. The limitations of acupuncture are discussed further in Chapter 7, entitled "Determining Whether Acupuncture is the Treatment of Choice."

RESOLVING CULTURAL CONFLICTS

The idea of inserting needles into the human body without injecting anything or withdrawing a body fluid seems strange and pointless to most American medical scientists. It seems absurd that sticking a wire-like needle superficially into the skin of one part of the body could relieve pain in another part.

Many Americans suspect that acupuncture is mainly a type of hypnosis or faith-healing. There is good scientific evidence to the contrary, however.[7-10] Acupuncture is effective for treating animals not susceptible to hypnosis or faith healing.[11,12] One does not have to believe in acupuncture to be helped by it.

Thousands of years before American and European scientists discovered atoms, electrons, and electricity, the Chinese developed a concept of the entire universe as being in balance between *Yin* and *Yang* energy factors. They regarded the body as a microcosm which required a balance of *Yin* and *Yang* body energy to enjoy good health.[13] Each part of the body was thought of as another microcosm which required a balance of *Yin* and *Yang* energy to function properly.[14] They thought disease symptoms were caused by an imbalance of *Yin* and *Yang* in some part of the body. Such imbalance might be caused by injury or bacterial invasion. The goal of acupuncture treatment was to restore the balance of *Yin* and *Yang* in the afflicted part and the body as a whole.[15]

Yin and *Yang* may be roughly equated with negatively and positively charged electricity, but these concepts are much more elaborate and are discussed further in Chapter 4.

It is not necessary to accept Chinese philosophical concepts in order to learn acupuncture. Even if one concludes that the Chinese had the wrong reasons for selecting the acupuncture points to treat a specific disorder, we can use the formulas they have worked out over the centuries for relieving pain and disabilities in various parts of the body. Some understanding of Chinese acupuncture theory, however, is helpful for deciding which of the listed acupuncture points to choose under various circumstances.

The practice of acupuncture is based on theories of energy flow in the body and can be described as external treatment of internal disorders. The Chinese developed these theories and diagrammed meridians of energy transmission to and from vital organs of the body thousands of years ago. Like low-voltage electricity, these major channels of body energy transmission are invisible and are not present in cadavers. During many years of experimenting, the Chinese discovered that inserting sharp objects superficially at certain points on these meridians could relieve pain or improve the function of other specific parts of the body at some distance from these points. They had observed that needles inserted into these points produced a special sensation they called *Te-Chi* or energization. Insertion of needles at points in adjacent areas of the skin did not produce this sensation.

Our observations of referred pain transmitted along nerve pathways are consistent with acupuncture theory, but we are just beginning to acknowledge that bioelectricity is not entirely dependent on nerve fibers for its transmission. Modern knowledge of embryology helps explain that parts of the body which appear entirely separate from each other after birth have a history of common derivation and, therefore, a relationship which is not evident on ordinary physical examination. Modern electronic instruments enable us to locate acupuncture points precisely where the ancient Chinese showed them to be. These instruments measure electric resistance, which is lower at the acupuncture points than in the surrounding tissues. More information on these subjects is given in the chapters entitled, "Neurophysiologic Mechanisms in Acupuncture" and "Electro-acupuncture."

EMOTIONAL FACTORS

American theories of psychosomatic medicine describing a mechanism of emotionally triggered pathology are in some ways similar to Chinese theories of vital energy imbalance, although the terminology used is quite different. American physicians have documented physiologic changes in the body attributed to certain emotions.[16,17] Then they have analyzed the potential results of such changes on the functioning of various organs. By such methods it is possible to establish a relationship between emotions and somatic pathology. If we translate vigorous emotions as *Yang* vital energy, and depressive emotions as *Yin*, we can see the similarity between Chinese theories and our own.

In both mainland China and Taiwan, acupuncture is the main treatment for schizophrenia and other forms of mental illness.[18] It is used instead of drugs and shock treatments but is not considered a substitute for psychotherapy. Addictions, anxiety, depression, and insomnia are especially responsive to acupuncture.[19,20] These conditions are being treated at the Washington Acupuncture Center and elsewhere. Even cases of schizophrenia have been treated successfully by acupuncture in the United States.[21]

Since psychotropic drugs have been found to damage the basal ganglia of the brain and impair the function of other vital organs, acupuncture could be a safe substitute for them in many cases. The author's experience in treating depression during the past fifteen years indicates that acupuncture gives more rapid and lasting relief than electro-convulsive therapy or antidepressant drugs. Other psychiatrists have reached similar conclusions.[22]

ACUPUNCTURE RESEARCH

Much more research is needed to evaluate the results of acupuncture in America and to reconcile the theories and practices of acupuncture with western medical knowledge. Unfortunately, double-blind experiments are not appropriate for acupuncture evaluation because patients can easily tell whether the needles have been inserted into acupuncture points or elsewhere.

Since the degree of skill an acupuncturist has makes a big difference in determining whether acupuncture is successful or not, much so-called "acupuncture research" in the United States has only demonstrated that the people inserting needles for experiments were not skilled acupuncturists. Having people without much training or experience in acupuncture fail to obtain good results from inserting needles in what they think are acupuncture points does not prove that acupuncture is ineffective. Too many studies of this type have been published in American medical journals. Only highly skilled acupuncturists should be used in clinical research to evaluate the effectiveness of acupuncture.

Another type of research for evaluating the results of acupuncture could be done on matched groups of patients who were all examined before and after treatment by physicians not employed by any organization giving acupuncture or other type of treatment with which it was to be compared.

Basic research to explain precisely how and why acupuncture works is being conducted at many institutions in North America, Europe, and Asia.[23-26] This is discussed further in Chapter 5.

The efforts of the Washington Acupuncture Center to develop protocols for clinical research and to evaluate the effects of acupuncture treatment of various conditions are described in Chapter 10.

LEGAL STATUS OF ACUPUNCTURE

Instead of welcoming acupuncture as a valuable addition to the modalities of medical treatment available for helping patients, some organizations and states have tried to outlaw it. Before many licensed physicians had had a chance to learn how to perform it, the District of Columbia passed a law in 1974 ruling that only licensed physicians and dentists could insert acupuncture needles. In April 1975, however, this law was declared unconstitutional.[27]

Most states have laws stating that acupuncture can be performed only under the direct supervision of a licensed physician. It is

hoped that all states will soon have procedures for examining and certifying acupuncturists who are not licensed physicians. They could
have a status similar to that of registered nurses or medical technicians. In 1974, the author prepared a treatise on "Acupuncturist as a
New Health Occupation" at the request of the American Medical Association's Committee on Emerging Health Manpower. This is included
in Chapter 11.

REFERENCES FOR CHAPTER 1

1. Bache, F. "Cases Illustrative of the Remedial Effects of Acupunc-
    ture," *North American Medical and Surgical Journal* (1826):
    311–321.

2. Osler, William. *The Principles and Practice of Medicine.* editions
    1–8, New York: Appleton, 1892–1916.

3. Sjölund, Bengt; and Eriksson, Margareta. "Electro-Acupuncture
    and Endogenous Morphines." *Lancet* 2 (Nov. 1976): 1085.

4. Miller, Richard J. "The Potential of Endorphins." *Behavioral
    Medicine* (May 1979) 30–33.

5. Warren, Frank Z. *Freedom from Pain through Acupressure,* New
    York: Fell Publishing Company, 1977.

6. Gordon, T; Larson, C.P., Jr.; Prestwich, R. "Unexpected Cardiac
    Arrest During Anesthesia and Surgery." *Journal of the American
    Medical Association,* 236 (1976): 2758–60.

7. Collison, D. "Acupuncture and Hynotherapy.", *Medical Journal
    of Australia* 2(3) (July 1974): 112.

8. Nemerof, Henry; and Rothman, Irwin. "Acupuncture and
    Hypnotism." *American Journal of Clinical Hypnosis* 16 (3)
    (January 1974): 156–159.

9. Frost, E.A. "Acupuncture and Hypnosis. Apples and Oranges.
    New York State Journal of Medicine, 78 (11) (September 1978):
    1768–72.

10. Mac Hovec, F.J.; and Man, S.C. "Acupuncture and Hypnosis
    Compared: Fifty-eight Cases." *American Journal of Clinical
    Hypnosis,* 21(1) (July 1978): 45–47.

11. Freeman, A. "Veterinary Acupuncture." *Journal of the
    American Veterinary Medicine Association* 164(5) (March 1,
    1974): 446–48.

12. Kao, F.F.; and Kao, J.J. "Veterinary Acupuncture." *American Journal of Chinese Medicine* 2(1) (January 1974): 89–102.

13. *Huang Ti Nei Ching Su Wen,* compiled *circa* 2600 B.C., Translated by Ilza Veith. *The Yellow Emperor's Classic of Internal Medicine,* Berkeley: University of California Press, 1949.

14. *Zhen Jiu Jia Yi Jing, A Classic of Acupuncture and Moxibustion,* including charts and colored diagrams of meridians and acupuncture points. Hong Kong: The Academy Press, Kowloon, 1964.

15. Hua, Shou, *Shi Si Jing Fa Huei* (In Chinese, first published *circa* 1300 B.C.) Peking: People's Hygiene Press, 1968.

16. Alexander, Franz; French T.M.; and Pollock G.H. *Psychosomatic Specificity, Experimental Study and Results,* vol. 1. Chicago: University of Chicago Press, 1968.

17. Lewis, Howard R.: and Lewis, Martha. *Psychosomatics.* New York: Viking, 1972.

18. Leseth, Knut. "Psychiatry in China." *Tidsskrift for den Norske Laegeforeining* 94(7) (10 March 1974): 439–441.

19. Chien, E.Y.; and Zakaria, S. "Acupuncture for Psychiatric Disorders." *Journal of the American Medical Association* 229(6) (August 5, 1974): 639.

20. Bresler, David E., *et al.* "The Potential of Acupuncture for the Behavioral Sciences." *American Psychologist* 30(3) (March 1975): 411–414.

21. Kane, Jonathan; and Di Scipio, William J. "Acupuncture Treatment of Schizophrenia." *American Journal of Psychiatry,* 136(3) (March 1979): 297–302.

22. Ullet, George A. Acupuncture: Pricking the Bubble of Skepticism." *Biological Psychiatry* 13(2) (April 1978): 159–161.

23. Liao, S.J. "Recent Advances in the Understanding of Acupuncture." *Yale Journal of Biological Medicine* 51(1) (January-February 1978): 55–65.

24. Mendelson, G. "The Possible Role of Enkephalin in the Mechanism of Acupuncture Analgesia in Man." *Medical Hypotheses* 2(4) (July–August 1977): 144–145.

25. McLennan, H.; Gilfillan K.; and Heap, Y. "Some Pharmacological Observations on the Analgesia Induced by Acupuncture in Rabbits." *Pain* 3(3) (June 1977): 229–238.

26.   Sjolund, B.; Terenius L.; and Eriksson, M. "Increased Cerebro-
      spinal Fluid Levels of Endorphins after Electro-acupuncture."
      Acta Physiologica Scandinavica 100(3) (July 1977): 382–384.

27.   Wensel v. Washington. *Law Review*. April 13, 1975 (CA 1004–74,
      Superior Court of the District of Columbia).

chapter 2

CLASSICAL MERIDIANS AND THEIR ACUPUNCTURE POINTS

Precise location of acupuncture points is crucial for obtaining the maximum therapeutic effect. This is difficult because of the differences in sizes and shapes of patients' bodies. Each acupuncture point is considered to be only about three millimeters in diameter.

Traditional Chinese acupuncturists spend years of training to learn the art of point location. Electronic point-finding instruments make this task much easier than it used to be. The point-finding instruments, however, only indicate the location of an acupuncture point without identifying which one it is. The acupuncturist must know which point he is looking for and its general location. Three-dimensional manikins with meridians and points clearly labeled in English greatly facilitate point location. Acupuncture students can map the points on each others' bodies with washable ink.

Most of the ancient Chinese textbooks depict acupuncture points on bodies with overly plump abdomens and short legs. However, using a system of body inches referred to as *cun* (*tsun* in earlier texts), these points can be identified on bodies of different proportions.

CHINESE BODY MEASUREMENT

The traditional methods of point localization are in units of measurement called *cun* and *fen*. A *cun* is approximately one inch in the average adult male. A *fen* is one-tenth of a *cun*. A *cun* is proportionate to body size and is, therefore, larger on large bodies than on smaller ones. A person whose legs are longer than average in proportion to his torso will have longer body *cun* on his legs than on his torso.

This system of body measurement is subject to considerable variation and is much less precise than point location with electric instruments. It is mainly useful to give a general idea of where points are when combined with knowledge of how to identify specific anatomical landmarks. Point location is actually an art more than a science or mathematical process. Years of locating acupuncture points on bodies of different sizes and shapes usually gives an acupuncturist the ability to locate them without consciously measuring or using any kind of instrument. Apparently, there is no substitute for experience in mastering this art.

In general, a *cun* is the width of the widest part of the thumb. In this system, anatomical landmarks are utilized to obtain units of length and width for each area on the body surface. Thus, a length between two anatomical landmarks, such as the distance from the wrist to the elbow, is the same number of *cun* regardless of the size of the body. Although an adult's arm is much longer than a child's in centimeters, both measure twelve *cun* from wrist to elbow.

The following measurements in *cun* are listed in most books on acupuncture.

Cranial Cun.   The distance from the center of a line drawn through the supraorbital ridges to the depression on the posterior aspect of the skull is 15 *cun*. The distance between the posterior aspect of the mastoid processes of the skull is 9 *cun*.

Facial Cun.   From the center of the frontal eminence to the center of the mental protuberance of the chin is 10 *cun*. The distance between the lateral margins of the zygomatic bones across the anterior surface of the face is 7 *cun*.

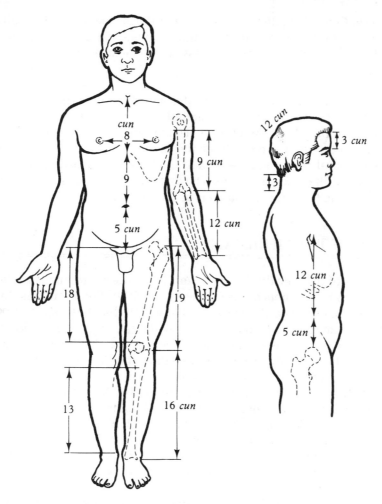

Figure 2–1.   Body measurement in cun for acupuncture

Anterior Chest and Abdominal Cun.   The distance from the mid-axillary fossa to the inferior margin of the eleventh rib is 12 cun. The distance from the xyphoid-sternal junction to the umbilicus is 8 cun. The distance between the nipples in men and children is 8 cun.

Back cun.   The distance between the vertebral spaces in the thoracic spine is 1 cun. With the hands on opposite elbows, the distance from the medial margin of the scapula to the center of the vertebral column is 3 cun.

Arm Cun.   The distance from the anterior aspect of the axillary skin crease to the center of the cubital crease is 9 *cun*. The distance from the center of the cubital crease to the most distal crease of the wrist is 12 *cun*.

Leg Cun.   The distance from the superior pubic margin on the medial aspect of the thigh to the medial epicondyle of the femur is 18 *cun*. The distance from the greater trochanter on the lateral aspect of the thigh to the lateral condyle of the femur is 19 *cun*. The distance from the medial condyle of the tibia at the knee to the medial malleolus of the tibia at the ankle is 13 *cun*. The distance from the lateral condyle of the femur to the lateral malleolus of the fibula is 16 *cun*.

NOMENCLATURE OF THE MERIDIANS

The names of the meridians have been translated into English in various ways to relate them to the Chinese concept of the meridians' functions and the organs or body systems to which they have special relationships. Some of these names are misleading, quaint, or meaningless. The organs after which meridians are named do not seem to be involved in the etiology or pathology of the conditions treated by using acupuncture points on their meridians. Thus, the effectiveness of points on the gall bladder meridian is not altered by the removal of the patient's gall bladder. Points on the gall bladder meridian are useful for treating a variety of medical problems which seem unrelated to it. Some body structures, such as joints and muscles most commonly treated by acupuncture, have no meridian names. Acupuncture points for treating problems in these areas are on various meridians whose names seem unrelated to the problem or area being treated.

The meridians are mainly located in different parts of the body from the organs after which they were named. Thus, lung and heart meridian points are predominantly on the arms; many points of the gall bladder, urinary bladder, small intestine, colon, and stomach meridians are found on the head; the spleen and liver meridians are located mostly on the legs; and the colon meridian is not on the abdomen at all. These meridian organ names are retained for identification purposes because they have been used in most books written on acupuncture in the past.

Quaint meridian names, such as "triple warmer," "conception vessel," "heart governor," and "governing vessel," have been translated as "metabolism," "sex," "vascular," and "brain," respectively. These terms seem better translations of the Chinese into modern English.

Some acupuncture textbooks in English and other European

languages use letters of the alphabet or Roman numerals to label the meridians. There is a confusing amount of variation and no uniformity in the sequences different authors use.

Some Chinese books on acupuncture show diagrams of extensions of the meridians into deep body structures, connecting the meridians to the organs after which they were named. These internal connections, however, do not seem to serve any practical purpose in determining which acupuncture points to use for treating various medical problems. Although there is uniformity in almost all Chinese textbooks for diagrams of the classical meridians and their acupuncture points on the body surface, there is considerable variation in diagrams of the course of meridians inside the body. It seems pointless, therefore, to include such diagrams in this book.

The Chinese have different names for each acupuncture point. These names do not give clues as to on which meridian or on which part of the body the point is located. Neither do they indicate the potential therapeutic purpose for which the point might be used. These Chinese acupuncture point names seem somewhat like the names of towns on a geographical map and have little if any medical significance. A list of these names can be found in Appendix II. It seems more appropriate for Americans to learn to use numbers for each point on each meridian. Fortunately, there is uniformity in these numbers, as diagrammed in various American and European books and articles on acupuncture.

PRECISE LOCATION OF POINTS

The acupuncture points given in this chapter were designated by Chinese acupuncturists working at the Washington Acupuncture Center and verified with electronic instruments. They are similar to the points described and diagrammed in acupuncture textbooks for thousands of years.

Students should familiarize themselves with the general course of the meridians and with the location of acupuncture points on three-dimensional manikins as well as locating them on flat diagrams. It is necessary to have detailed knowledge of the location of large superficial blood vessels and other anatomic structures to avoid accidentally piercing them with acupuncture needles. It is especially important to avoid insertion of needles into the pleural cavity, the heart, the spinal cord, the eye, the nasal sinuses, or the abdominal viscera. Beginning students should have diagrams of these structures in front of them while attempting to locate acupuncture points. Acupuncture needles should not be inserted without knowing precisely what structures are being pierced.

Meridian Lu (Lung, Shou Tai Yin Fei Ching, Hand–Taiyin, A)

There are 11 acupuncture points on the Lung Meridian (LU), which begins above the axilla on the chest and descends down the arm to the thumb. (See Figure 2–2).

Lu 1   (*Chungfu, Zhongfu*): 1 cun below the clavicle at the midclavicular line, in the interspace between the first and second ribs; perpendicularly, 3 to 5 *fen* beneath the skin surface.

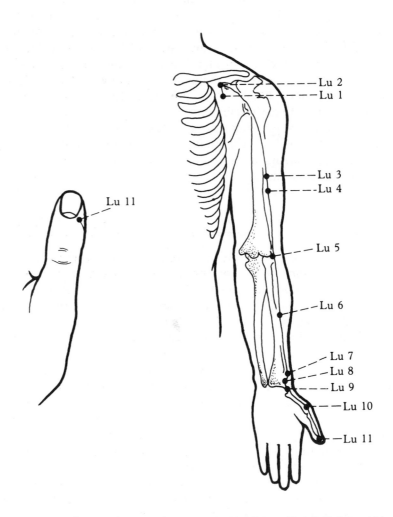

Figure 2–2.   Meridian Lu (Lung, *Shou Tai Yin Fei* Ching, Hand–*Taiyin*, A)

Lu 2   (*Yunmen*): In the triangular depression on the inferior margin of the coracoclavicular ligament, 1 *cun* above Lu 1; perpendicularly, 3 to 5 *fen*.

Lu 3   (*Tianfu*): On the medial aspect of the upper arm, 3 *cun* below the anterior axillary fold, on the radial side of the biceps muscle, 6 *cun* above Lu 5; perpendicularly, 4 to 9 *fen*.

Lu 4   (*Xiabai*): On the medial aspect of the upper arm, anterolateral to the humerus bone, about 2 *cun* directly below Lu 3; perpendicularly, 4 to 9 *fen*.

Lu 5   (*Chize*): On the lateral aspect of the tendon of the biceps brachii muscle in the cubital crease with the elbow rotated slightly medially; perpendicularly, 5 to 9 *fen*.

Lu 6   (*Kungtsui, Kongzui*): Connect a line between Lu 5 and Lu 9. Lu 6 is located on the medial border of the radius, 7 *cun* from Lu 9 and 5 *cun* from Lu 5; perpendicularly, 5 to 9 *fen*.

Lu 7   (*Liehchueh, Lieque*): 1.5 *cun* above the most distal wrist crease, above the styloid process of the radius on the volar surface of the arm; obliquely, 5 to 9 *fen*.

Lu 8   (*Jingqu*): One *cun* above the transverse fold of the wrist on the medial side of the styloid process of the radius bone; perpendicularly, 2 to 4 *fen*, avoiding the radial artery.

Lu 9   (*Taiyuan*): On the inferior margin of the lateral aspect of the greater multiangular carpal bone at the pulse point, perpendicularly, 2 to 3 *fen*, being careful not to pierce the radial artery.

Lu 10 (*Yuchi, Yuji*): Over the middle of the first metacarpal bone on palmar surface; perpendicularly, 3 to 6 *fen*.

Lu 11 (*Shaoshang*): On the radial aspect of the thumb about one *fen* from the nail bed, perpendicularly, 2 to 4 *fen*.

Meridian Co (Colon, Shou Yang Min Ta Chang Ching, Hand–Yangming, B)

There are 20 acupuncture points on Meridian Co, which begins on the index finger and extends upward via the lateral aspect of the arm to the face. (See Figure 2–3.)

Co 1   (*Shangyang*): At the radial aspect of the third digit about 1 *fen* below the nail base of the third finger, just under the skin.

Co 2   (*Erhchien, Erjian*): On the dorsum of the hand, on the radial aspect at the metacarpal phalangeal joint of the third finger, perpendicularly 3 *fen*.

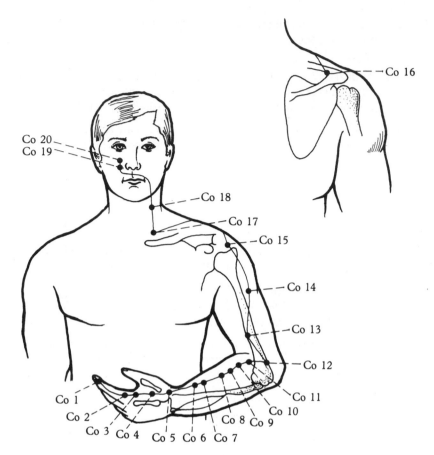

Figure 2-3.   Meridian Co (Colon, *Shou Yang Ming Ta Chang Ching*, Hand–Yangming, B)

Co 3   (*Sanchien, Sanjian*): On the dorsum of the hand, on the radial aspect of the distal end of the metacarpal bone of the index finger, with the fist slightly closed, insert needle perpendicularly 3 to 7 *fen*.

Co 4   (*Hoku, Hegu*): On the dorsum of the hand between the first and second metacarpal bones over the protuberance of the muscle on the radial side in the middle of the second metacarpal bone, insert needle perpendicularly, 3 to 7 *fen*. (Do not use on a pregnant woman.)

Co 5   (*Yangshi, Yangxi*): On the dorsal surface of the hand overlying the scaphoid navicular bone between the tendon of the extensor pollicis brevis and extensor pollicis longus, perpendicularly, 3 to 5 *fen*.

Co 6 (*Peinli, Pianli*): 3 *cun* above Co 5 on the line connecting Co 5 and Co 11, insert needle perpendicularly, 3 to 5 *fen*.

Co 7 (*Wenliu*): 5 *cun* above Co 5 on the line connecting Co 5 and Lu 11, perpendicularly, 3 to 8 *fen*.

Co 8 (*Xialian*): 4 *cun* below Co 11, perpendicularly, 3 to 8 *fen*.

Co 9 (*Shanglian*): 3 *cun* below Co 11, perpendicularly, 3 to 8 *fen*.

Co 10 (*Shousanli*): 2 *cun* below Co 11 on the medial aspect of the radius, insert needle perpendicularly, 8 *fen* to 1.2 *cun*.

Co 11 (*Quchi*): In the depression at the lateral end of the transverse cubital crease, midway between Lu 5 and the lateral epicondyle of the humerus, when the elbow is half flexed, insert needle perpendicularly, 6 *fen* to 1.2 *cun*.

Co 12 (*Zhouliao*): Over the lateral epicondyle of the humerus on the lateral border of the humerus, perpendicularly, 8 *fen* to 1 *cun*.

Co 13 (*Wuli*): On the antero-medial border of the humerus, 3 *cun* above the elbow crease, perpendicularly, 8 *fen* to 1.2 *cun*, being careful to avoid the brachial artery.

Co 14 (*Binao*): At the lower border of the deltoid muscle insertion into the humerus in line with Co 11 and Co 15, perpendicularly, 2 to 5 *fen*.

Co 15 (*Chienyu, Jianyu*): On the inferior margin of the acromial process at the articulation of the shoulder 2 *cun* below the posterior margin of the clavicle, insert needle perpendicularly, 6 *fen* to 1.5 *cun*.

Co 16 (*Jugu*): On the back in the depression between the clavicular-acromial extremity and the spine of the scapula, laterally oblique, 7 *fen* to 1 *cun*, being careful not to pierce the upper lobe of the lung.

Co 17 (*Tianding*): About 1 *cun* below Co 18 at the posterior border of the sterno-cleido-mastoid muscle when the patient is sitting straight with his head erect, perpendicularly, 3 to 8 *fen*.

Co 18 (*Neck–Futu*): 3 *cun* lateral to the thyroid cartilage on the posterior border of the sterno-cleido-mastoid muscle, perpendicularly, 2 to 6 *fen*, being careful to avoid major blood vessels in this area.

Co 19 (*Nose–Heliao*): 0.5 *cun* lateral to the nasolabial cleft midway between the nose and mouth, obliquely, 2 to 4 *fen*.

Co 20 (*Yinghsiang, Yingxiang*): At the central point of the anterior margin of the ala nasi and the nasolabial sulcus, insert needle 3 to 6 *fen*, obliquely.

Meridian St (Stomach, Tsu Yang Ming Wei Ching, Foot–Yangming, C)

There are 45 acupuncture points on the Stomach Meridian, which begins on the face and descends to the second toe. (See Figure 2–4.) The 23 most frequently used are:

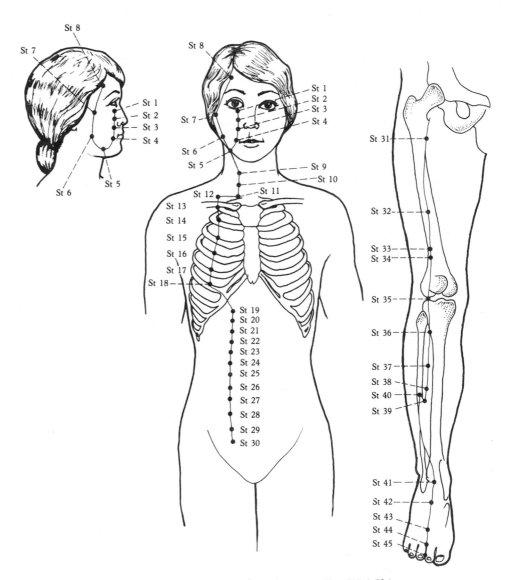

Figure 2–4. Meridian St (Stomach, Tsu Yang Ming Wei Ching, Foot–Yangming, C)

St 2   (*Szupai, Sibai*): In the middle of the infra-orbital foramen on the cheek, 5 to 8 *fen* superficially along the skin.

St 4   (*Titsang, Dicang*): Under St 2 and at a level of about 4 *fen* from the angle of the mouth inside the nasolabial sulcus, obliquely toward the cheek at a depth of 7 *fen* to 1 *cun*.

St 6   (*Chiache, Jiache*): About 4 *fen* above the angle of the mandible overlying the anterior muscle on the depression of that muscle, perpendicularly, 3 to 5 *fen*.

St 7   (*Hsiakuan, Xiaguan*): In the depression between the inferior border of the zygomatic arch and the mandibular notch, perpendicularly, 5 *fen*.

St 8   (*Touwei*): Overlying the frontal eminence, horizontally along the skin for 3 to 5 *fen* laterally.

St 21   (*Liangmen*): 2 *cun* laterally from the midline, 4 *cun* above the umbilicus, perpendicularly, 5 *fen* to 1 *cun*.

St 25   (*Tienshu*): 2 *cun* from the left and the right of the umbilicus, perpendicularly, 5 to 8 *fen*.

St 27   (*Tachu, Daju*): 2 *cun* from the left and the right of the median below the umbilicus or 2 *cun* below St 25, perpendicularly, 4 to 8 *fen*.

St 28   (*Shuitao, Shuidao*): 2 *cun* from the left and the right from Kuanyuan (Sx 4), which is 3 *cun* vertically below the umbilicus, perpendicularly, 5 to 8 *fen*.

St 31   (*Pikuan, Biguan*): Below the anterior superior spine of the ilium, in the depression on the lateral side of the sartorius muscle, with the thigh flexed, perpendicularly, 1 to 1.5 *cun*.

St 32   (*Futu, Femur-Futu*): 6 *cun* above the upper margin of the patella, along the line connecting the lateral margin of the patella and the anterior superior iliac spine, perpendicularly, 1 to 1.5 *cun*.

St 33   (*Yinshi*): 3 *cun* above the patella, along its lateral margin, perpendicularly 7 *fen* to 1 *cun*.

St 34   (*Liangchiu*): The location of St 34 (*Liangchiu*) is 2 *cun* above the superior margin of the patella with the knees flexed, perpendicularly, 7 *fen* to 1 *cun*.

St 35   (*Tupi, Dubi*): In the depression of the lateral aspect of the patellar ligament when the knee is flexed, obliquely to a depth of 7 *fen* to 1.2 *cun*.

St 36   (*Tsusanli, Zusanli*): 3 *cun* below the tuberosity of the tibia on the lateral aspect of the tibialis anterior muscle, 5 *fen* to 1.5 *cun* perpendicularly.

St 37   (*Shangchushu, Shangjuxu*): 6 *cun* below St 35 on the lateral aspect of the tibia, perpendicularly, 5 *fen* to 1.5 *cun*.

St 38   (*Tiaokou*): 8 *cun* below the knee, 2 *cun* below St 37, perpendicularly, 1 *cun*.

St 39   (*Hsiachushu, Xiajuxu*): 3 *cun* below St 37 and 9 *cun* below St 35, perpendicularly, 5 *fen* to 1 *cun*.

St 40   (*Fenglung*): 8 *cun* above the anterior aspect of the lateral malleolus, parallel to St 38 (*Tiaokou*) at a distance of 1 *cun*.

St 41   (*Chiehshi, Jiexi*): Over the dorsum of the foot, in the center of the cruciate crural ligament, between the tendons of the extensor hallucis longus and the extensor digitorum longus, perpendicularly toward the ankle to a depth of 5 to 7 *fen*.

St 43   (*Hsienku, Xiangu*): Between the second and the third metatarsal bones, 2 *cun* above St 44, perpendicularly, 5 to 7 *fen*.

St 44   (*Neiting*): In the interspace between the second and the third metatarsals between the bases of the second and third toes, perpendicularly, 5 to 7 *fen*.

St 45   (*Litui, Lidui*): About 1 *fen* from the lateral aspect of the angle of the vallum unguis of the second toe, obliquely to a depth of 1 *fen*.

Meridian Sp (Spleen, Tsu Tai Yin Pi Ching, Foot–Taiyin, D)

There are 21 acupuncture points on Meridian Sp (Figure 2–5). The 7 most frequently used are:

Sp 1   (*Yinpai, Yinbai*): About 1 *fen* medial to the base of the great toe, obliquely to a depth of 1 *fen*.

Sp 4   (*Kungsun, Gongsun*): 1 *cun* behind the proximal end of the proximal phalange on the medial aspect of the foot at the anterior inferior border of the distal end of the first metatarsal bone, perpendicularly, 7 to 9 *fen*.

Sp 5   (*Shangchiu*): In the depression at the anterior border under the medial malleolus, between the tibia and the talas, perpendicularly, 2 to 3 *fen*.

Sp 6   (*Sanyinchiao, Sanyinjiao*): 3 *cun* above the apex of the medial malleolus, behind the tibia, perpendicularly, 5 *fen* to 1 *cun* (not to be used in pregnant patients, except to facilitate delivery).

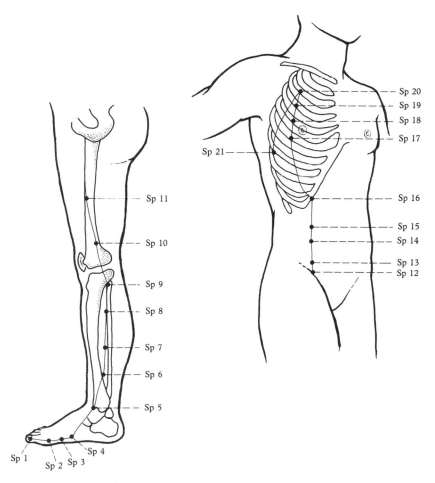

Figure 2–5.   Meridian Sp (Spleen, *Tsu Tai Yin Pi Ching*, Foot–*Taiyin*, D)

Sp 9   (*Yinlinchuan*): Under the medial condyle of the tibia, on the medial aspect below the knee, level with GB 34 (*Yanglinchuan*), perpendicularly, 5 *fen* to 1.5 *cun*.

Sp 10   (*Hsiehhai, Xuehai*): 2 *cun* above the medial border of the patella over the protuberance of the medial thigh, when the knee is flexed (from the upper border of the patella to the superior border of the pubic bone is 18 *cun*), perpendicularly, 7 *fen* to 1.2 *cun*.

Sp 15   (*Taheng, Daheng*): 3.5 to 4 *cun* above the umbilicus, along the lateral aspect of the rectus abdominis muscle, perpendicularly, 5 to 8 *fen*.

Meridian He (Heart, Shou Shao Yin Hsin Ching, Hand–Shaoyin, E)

There are 9 acupuncture points on Meridian He (Figure 2–6). The 7 most frequently used are:

He 3   (*Shaohai*): Overlying the medial epicondyle of the humerus with the arm flexed, perpendicularly, 5 to 10 *fen*.

He 4   (*Lingtao, Lingdao*): On the muscle flexor carpi ulnaris, vertically, downward 1.5 *cun*, level with the posterior margin of the capitulum ulnae or 1.5 *cun* above He 7 (*Shenmen*), perpendicularly, 3 to 5 *fen*.

He 5   (*Tungli, Tongli*): 1 *cun* below the pisiform bone and level with the center of the articular surface of the distal end of the ulna or 1 *cun* above He 7 (*Shenmen*), perpendicularly, 3 to 5 *fen*.

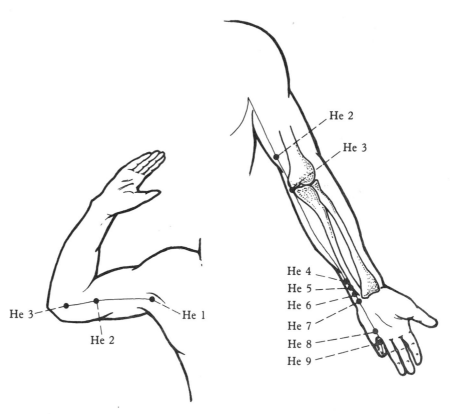

Figure 2–6.   Meridian He (Heart, *Shou Shao Yin Hsin Ching*, Hand–Shaoyin, E)

He 6 (*Yinhsi, Yinxi*): 5 *fen* from the posterior margin of the lateral aspect of the pisiform bone, level with the anterior margin of the articular surface of the distal end of the ulna or 0.5 *cun* above He 7 (*Shenmen*), perpendicularly, 3 to 5 *fen*.

He 7 (*Shenmen*): Along the most distal skin crease of the wrist on the ulnar side of the flexor carpi ulnaris muscle, perpendicularly, 3 to 5 *fen*.

He 8 (*Shaofu*): On the first skin crease on the palm between the fourth and fifth metacarpal bones, perpendicularly, 3 to 5 *fen*.

He 9 (*Shaochung, Shaochong*): About 1 *fen* from the base of the nail on the radial aspect of the fifth finger, obliquely to a depth of 1 *fen*.

Meridian SI (Small Intestine, Shou Tai Yang Hsiao Chang Ching, Hand–Taiyang, F)

There are 19 acupuncture points on Meridian SI (Figure 2–7). The 15 most frequently used are:

SI 1 (*Shaotse, Shaoze*): On the ulnar aspect of the fifth finger, about 1 *fen* from the base of the nail, obliquely to a depth of 1 *fen*.

SI 3 (*Houshi, Houxi*): On the ulnar aspect of the metacarpal–phalangeal joint of the fifth finger. This point is located laterally behind the end of the fifth metacarpal bone when the fist is slightly clenched, perpendicularly, 5 *fen* to 1 *cun*.

SI 4 (*Wanku, Hand–Wangu*): On the ulnar side of the hand between the fifth metacarpal bone and the hamate bone, perpendicularly, 3 to 5 *fen*.

SI 5 (*Yangku, Yanggu*): On the ulnar side of the ulnocarpal joint, between the styloid process of the ulna and the pisiform bone, perpendicularly, 3 to 5 *fen*.

SI 6 (*Yanglao*): On the radial aspect of the styloid process of the ulna, perpendicularly to a depth of 5 *fen* to 1 *cun*.

SI 7 (*Chihcheng, Zhizheng*): On the radial side, 5 *cun* above SI 5, perpendicularly 5 *fen* to 1 *cun*.

SI 8 (*Hsiaohai, Xiaohai*): In the fossa between the ulnar olecranon and the medial epicondyle of the humerus, with the elbow flexed, perpendicularly to a depth of 3 to 5 *fen*.

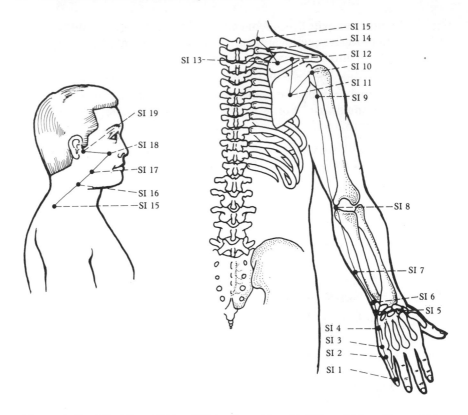

Figure 2–7.   Meridian SI (Small Intestine, *Shou Tai Yang Hsiao Chang Ching*, Hand–*Taiyang*, F)

SI 9   (*Chienchen, Jianzhen*): 1 *cun* above the posterior axillary fold, at the inferior posterior border of the shoulder joint, perpendicularly to a depth of 5 to 8 *fen*.

SI 10   (*Naoshu*): Above SI 9, in the depression below the spine of the scapula, perpendicularly to a depth of 5 to 8 *fen*.

SI 11   (*Tientsung, Tianzong*): Level with the spinuous process of the fourth thoracic vertebra, in the infraspinatous fossa, perpendicularly to a depth of 5 to 7 *fen*.

SI 12   (*Pingfeng, Bingfeng*): In the center of the suprascapular fossa, 1 *cun* above the center of the superior margin of the spine of the scapula (SI 12, SI 10, and SI 11 form a triangle), perpendicularly, 5 to 7 *fen*.

SI 14   (*Chienwaishu, Jianwaishu*): 3 *cun* from Br 13, below the spinous process of the first thoracic vertebra, obliquely to a depth of 3 to 6 *fen*.

SI 15   (*Chienchungshu, Jianzhongshu*): In the depression of the seventh cervical vertebra and 2 *cun* lateral to Br 14, obliquely to a depth of 3 to 6 *fen*.

SI 18   (*Chuanliao, Quanliao*): Directly below the external canthus in the depression below the lower border of the zygomatic bone, perpendicularly to a depth of 4 to 8 *fen*.

SI 19   (*Tingkung, Tinggong*): In the depression between the tragus and mandibular joint when the mouth is slightly opened, perpendicularly to a depth of 5 *fen* to 1 *cun*.

Meridian UB (Urinary Bladder, Tsu Tai Yang Pang Kuang Ching, Foot–Taiyang, G)

There are 67 acupuncture points on Meridian G (Figure 2–8). The 32 most frequently used are:

UB 1   (*Chingming, Jingming*): On the margin of the orbit and 1 *fen* below the inner canthus of the eye, perpendicularly to a depth of 2 *fen*, being very careful not to touch the eyeball. (This point is too close to the eye to be safe for the beginner to use.)

UB 2   (*Tsanchu, Zanzhu*): 1 *fen* into the margin of the medial end of the supraorbital margin (eyebrow), outward to a depth of 3 *fen*, being very careful not to touch the eyeball.

UB 11   (*Tachu, Dashu*): Lateral to the lower end of the spine of the first thoracic vertebra to a distance of 1.5 *cun* (from the medial line to the medial border of the scapula is 3 *cun*), obliquely to a depth of 3 *fen*.

UB 12   (*Fengmen*): In the depression, 1.5 *cun* lateral to the lower border of the spinous process of the second thoracic vertebra, obliquely to a depth of 3 to 5 *fen*.

UB 13   (*Feishu*): In the depression 1.5 *cun* lateral to the third thoracic vertebra, downward and obliquely, 3 to 5 *fen*.

UB 15   (*Hsinshu, Xinshu*): In the depression, 1.5 *cun* lateral to the fifth thoracic vertebra, obliquely, 3 to 5 *fen*.

UB 17   (*Keshu, Geshu*): In the depression, 1.5 *cun* lateral to the seventh thoracic vertebra, downward and obliquely, 3 to 5 *fen*.

UB 18   (*Kanshu, Ganshu*): In the depression, 1.5 *cun* lateral to the lower border of the spinous process of the ninth thoracic vertebra, perpendicularly, 3 to 5 *fen*.

UB 19   (*Tanshu, Danshu*): In the depression, 1.5 *cun* lateral to the lower border of the spinous process of the tenth thoracic vertebra, downward and obliquely, 3 to 5 *fen*.

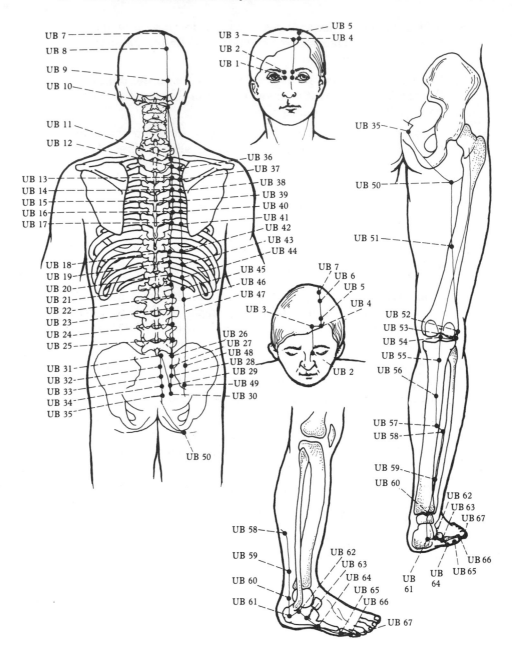

Figure 2–8. Meridian UB (Urinary Bladder, *Tsu Tai Yang Pang Kuang Ching*, Foot–*Taiyang*, G)

UB 20 (*Pishu*): In the depression, 1.5 *cun* lateral to the lower border of the spinous process of the first thoracic vertebra, downward and obliquely, 3 to 5 *fen*.

UB 21 (*Weishu*): In the depression, 1.5 *cun* lateral to the lower border of the spinous process of the twelfth thoracic vertebra, obliquely, 3 to 5 *fen*.

UB 22 (*Sanchiaoshu, Sanjiaoshu*): In the depression, 1.5 *cun* lateral to the lower border of the spinous process of the first lumbar vertebra, perpendicularly, 3 to 5 *fen*.

UB 23 (*Shenshu*): In the depression, 1.5 *cun* lateral to the lower border of the spinous process of the second lumbar vertebra, perpendicularly, 5 *fen* to 1 *cun*.

UB 25 (*Tachangshu, Dachangshu*): In the depression, 1.5 *cun* lateral to the lower border of the spinous process of the fourth lumbar vertebra, perpendicularly, 7 *fen* to 1 *cun*.

UB 26 (*Kuanguanshu, Guanguanshu*): In the depression, 1.5 *cun* lateral to the lower border of the spinous process of the fifth lumbar vertebra, perpendicularly, 7 *fen* to 1 *cun*.

UB 27 (*Hsiaochangshu, Xiaochangshu*): In the depression, 1.5 *cun* lateral to the midline of the back at the level of the first posterior sacral foramen, perpendicularly, 5 *fen* to 1.5 *cun*.

UB 28 (*Pankuangshu, Pangguangshu*): In the depression, 1.5 *cun* lateral to the midline between the lower medial border of the posterior superior iliac spine and the sacrum, perpendicularly, 5 *fen* to 1.5 *cun*.

UB 31 (*Shangliao*): On the first posterior sacral foramen and about midway between the posterior superior iliac spine and the midline, 5 to 7 *fen* perpendicularly.

UB 32 (*Tzuliao, Ciliao*): On the second posterior sacral foramen and midway between the lower border of the posterior superior iliac spine and the median line, 5 to 7 *fen* perpendicularly.

UB 33 (*Chungliao, Zhongliao*): On the third posterior sacral foramen between UB 29 and the midline, 5 to 7 *fen* perpendicularly.

UB 34 (*Hsialiao, Xialiao*): On the fourth posterior sacral foramen between UB 30 and the midline, 5 to 7 *fen* perpendicularly.

UB 38 (*Kaohuang, Fuxi*): In the depression, 3 *cun* lateral to the fourth thoracic vertebra, obliquely, 3 to 5 *fen*.

UB 47 (*Chihshih*): In the depression, 3 *cun* from the left and the right sides of the second lumbar vertebra, perpendicularly, 7 *fen* to 1.5 *cun*.

UB 49   (*Chihpien*): In the depression, 3 *cun* from the left and the right sides of the fourth sacral vertebra, perpendicularly, 5 *fen* to 1 *cun*.

UB 50   (*Chengfu*): In the middle of the upper border of the thigh just below the buttocks, perpendicularly, 7 *fen* to 1 *cun*.

UB 51   (*Yenmen*) 6 *cun* below UB 50 (*Chengfu*) and in the center of the back of the thigh, perpendicularly, 5 *fen* to 1 *cun*.

UB 54   (*Weichung*): In the center of the popliteal fossa, perpendicularly, 5 *fen* to 1 *cun*.

UB 57   (*Chengshan*): Below the protuberance of the gastrocnemius muscle, midway between UB 54 (*Weichung*) and the upper border of the heel, perpendicularly, 5 *fen* to 1.5 *cun*.

UB 58   (*Feiyang*): 7 *cun* above UB 60 (*Kunlun*) at the lateral aspect of the gastrocnemius muscle, perpendicularly 5 *fen* to 1 *cun*.

UB 60   (*Kunlun*): In the depression lateral to the tendo calcaneus behind the lateral malleolus, perpendicularly, 5 *fen* to 8 *fen*.

UB 62   (*Shenmo, Shenmai*): In the depression, 5 *fen* below the inferior margin of the lateral malleolus, perpendicularly, 3 to 5 *fen*.

UB 67   (*Chihyin, Zhiyin*): About 1 *fen* lateral to the base of the nail of the fifth toe, obliquely, 1 to 3 *fen*. (Do not use on pregnant women, except to facilitate delivery.)

Meridian Ki (Kidney, Tsu Shao Yin Sheng Ching, Foot–Shaoyin, H)

There are 27 points on Meridian Ki (Figure 2–9). The 7 most frequently used are:

Ki 1   (*Yungchuan, Yongquan*): In the depression present when the toes are flexed, on the sole, in the center of the transverse arch, perpendicularly, 5 to 8 *fen*.

Ki 2   (*Janku, Rangu*): In the depression on the inferior border of the tuberosity of the navicular bone, perpendicularly, 8 *fen* to 1 *cun*.

Ki 3   (*Taihsi, Taixi*): In the depression directly below the medial malleolus, perpendicularly, 8 *fen* to 1.2 *cun*.

Ki 4   (*Tachung, Dazhong*): On the level of the inferior medial malleolus and beside the tendo calcaneus, perpendicularly, 3 to 5 *fen*.

Ki 6   (*Chaohai, Zhaohai*): In the depression above the heel, behind the medial malleolus, perpendicularly, 7 *fen* to 1 *cun*.

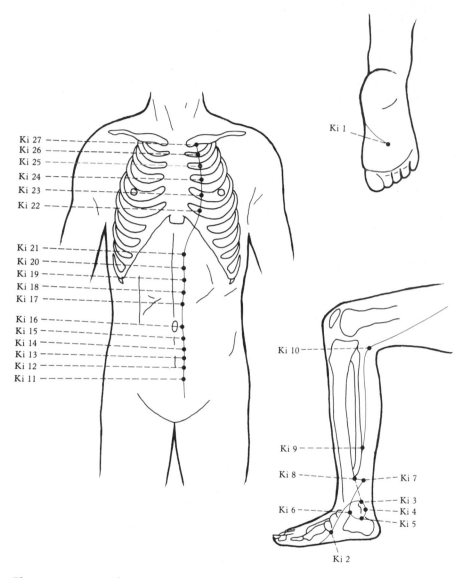

Figure 2-9. Meridian Ki (Kidney, *Tsu Shao Yin Sheng Ching*, Foot–Shaoyin, H)

Ki 7   (*Fuliu*): 2 *cun* above the posterior aspect of the medial malleolus, perpendicularly, 5 *fen* to 1 *cun*.

Ki 10   (*Yinku, Yingu*): At the medial aspect of the popliteal fossa, between the semitendinosus muscle and the semimembranosus muscle when the knee is flexed, perpendicularly, 8 *fen* to 1 *cun*.

Meridian Va (Vascular, Shou Chueh Yin Hsin Pao Ching, Hand–Jueyin, Circulation, I Pericardium, P)

There are 9 acupuncture points on Meridian Va (Figure 2–10). The 7 most frequently used are:

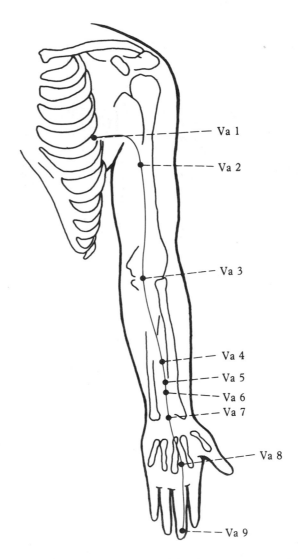

Figure 2–10. Meridian Va (Vascular, *Shou Chueh Yin Hsin Pao Ching*, Hand–Jueyin, Circulation, I Pericardium, P)

Va 3   (*Chutse, Quze*): In the middle of the elbow crease at the medial aspect of the tendons of the biceps brachii muscle, perpendicularly, 5 to 8 *fen*.

Va 4   (*Hsimen, Ximen*): In the center of the volar surface of the forearm 5 *cun* above the base of the palm, perpendicularly, 5 *fen* to 1 *cun*.

Va 5   (*Chienshih, Jianshi*): 3 *cun* above Va 7 in between the tendons of the palmaris longus muscle and the flexor carpi radialis muscle, perpendicularly, 8 *fen* to 1.3 *cun*.

Va 6   (*Neikuan, Neiguan*): 2 *cun* above Va 7 in between the palmaris longus muscle and the flexor carpi radialis muscle, perpendicularly, 5 *fen* to 1 *cun*.

Va 7   (*Taling, Daling*): In the middle of the most distal skin crease of the wrist in between the two tendons of the palmaris longus muscle and the flexor carpi radialis muscle, perpendicularly, 3 to 5 *fen*.

Va 8   (*Laokung, Laogong*): Between the second and the third metacarpal bones, where the tip of the middle finger touches when the fist is clenched, perpendicularly, 5 to 8 *fen*.

Va 9   (*Chungchung, Zhongchong*): About 1 *fen* from the tip of the volar aspect of the middle finger, perpendicularly, 2 *fen*.

Meridian Me (Metabolism, Shou Shao Yang San Chiao Ching, Sanjiao, Hand–Shaoyang, Triple Warmer, J)

There are 23 acupuncture points on Meridian Me (Figure 2–11). The 11 most frequently used are:

Me 1   (*Kuangchung, Guanchong*): About 1 *fen* proximal from the base of the nail on the ulnar aspect of the fourth digit, obliquely to a depth of 2 *fen*.

Me 2   (*Yemen*): On the back of the hand behind the web of the fourth and the fifth digit and in front of the metacarpal phalangeal joint, perpendicularly, 5 to 8 *fen*.

Me 3   (*Chungchu, Zhongzhu*): Between the fourth and fifth metacarpal bones, about 1 *cun* proximal from *Yemen*, perpendicularly, 5 to 8 *fen*.

Me 4   (*Yangchi*): Near the center of the skin crease on the dorsum of the wrist, at the ulnar aspect of the extensor digitorum communis muscle, perpendicularly, 3 *fen*.

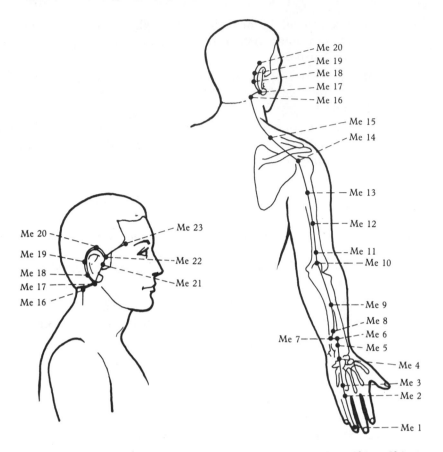

Figure 2-11.   Meridian Me (Metabolism, *Shou Shao Yang San Chiao Ching,* *Sanjiao* Hand–*Shaoyang,* Triple Warmer, J)

Me 5   (*Waikuan, Waiguan*): 2 *cun* above the skin crease on the dorsum of the wrist between the ulna and the radius, 5 *fen* to 1 *cun* perpendicularly.

Me 6   (*Chihkou, Zhigou*): 2 *cun* above the skin crease on the dorsum of the wrist between the ulna and radius, 5 *fen* to 1 *cun* perpendicularly.

Me 7   (*Huitsung, Huizong*): In the depression, 1 finger width behind the upper part of the olecranon with the elbow slightly flexed, 3 to 5 *fen* perpendicularly.

Me 14   (*Chienliao, Jianliao*): At the posterior inferior site of the acromion, level with Co 15, obliquely, 5 *fen* to 1 *cun*.

Me 17   (*Yifeng*): Behind the lobule of the auricle, in the depression between the mastoid process and the mandible, perpendicularly to a depth of 5 *fen* to 1 *cun*. (This depth is recommended by Chinese textbooks, but considering possible damage to the middle ear ossicles and the superficiality of the carotid artery, use of this point should be avoided or the needles only inserted 2 to 3 millimeters in the U.S.)

Me 21 (*Erhem, Ermen*): At the front of the tuberculum supratragicum, near the margin of the bone, where a depression is formed when the mouth is opened, perpendicularly, 3 to 5 *fen*.

Me 23 (*Szuchukung, Sizhukong*): At the lateral end of the supraorbital margin, superficially posteriorly 2 to 3 *fen*. (This point is too close to the eye for the beginner to use.)

Meridian GB (Gall Bladder, Tsu Shao Yang Tan Ching, Foot–Shaoyang, K)

There are 44 acupuncture points on Meridian GB (Figure 2–12). The 15 most frequently used are:

GB 1   (*Tungtzuliao, Tongziliao*): 5 *fen* lateral to the external canthus, outwardly and horizontally 5 to 8 *fen*, being careful not to touch the eye with a needle.

GB 2   (*Tinghui*): On the posterior margin of the condyloid process of the mandible, in front of the incisura intertragica, where a depression is formed when the mouth is wide open, perpendicularly, 6 *fen* to 1 *cun*.

GB 14 (*Yangpai, Yangbai*): 1 *cun* above the eyebrow, in the depression on the superciliary arch, downward to a depth of 3 to 5 *fen*, being very careful not to touch the eyeball.

GB 20 (*Fengchi*): From the median line of the back of the neck, upward 1 *cun* into the natural hairline, form a line with the inferior margin of the mastoid process behind the ear. In the middle of that line is GB 20 (*Fengchi*), in the depression beside the trapezoid muscle, 3 to 5 *fen* perpendicularly.

GB 21 (*Chienchin, Jianjing*): In the middle of a line from the seventh cervical vertebra to the acromion downward toward the nipples, perpendicularly, 3 to 5 *fen*.

GB 26 (*Taimo, Daimai*): At the level of the umbilicus, on the midaxillary line, 5 *fen* to 1 *cun* perpendicularly.

GB 29 (*Chuliao, Femur–Juliao*): On the iliac aspect between the anterior superior iliac spine and the greater trochanter of the femur, perpendicularly, 6 *fen* to 1 *cun*.

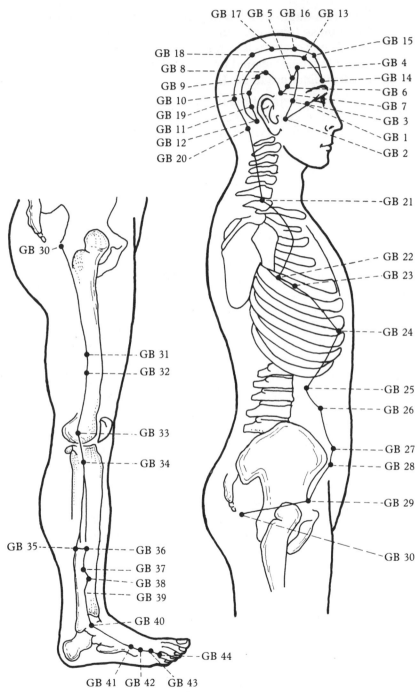

Figure 2–12.   Meridian GB (Gall Bladder, *Tsu Shao Yang Tan Ching*, Foot–*Shaoyang*, K)

GB 30 (*Huantiao*): On the posterior superior aspect of the greater trochanter one–third the distance, posteriorly, from the greater trochanter to the sacral hiatus 1.5 to 2.5 *cun* perpendicularly.

GB 31 (*Fengshi*): On the lateral aspect of the thigh, 7 *cun* above the patella (from the greater trochanter to the knee point is 19 *cun*), 1 to 1.5 *cun* perpendicularly.

GB 33 (*Yangkuan, Xiyangguan*): 3 *cun* above GB 34 (*Yanglinchuan*) in the depression above the lateral condyle of the femur, 5 to 8 *fen* perpendicularly.

GB 34 (*Yanglingchuan*): On the anterior inferior aspect of the capitulum of the fibula, 2 *cun* below the knee, 8 *fen* to 1.5 *cun* perpendicularly.

GB 37 (*Kuangming, Guangming*): 5 *cun* above the lateral malleolus in front of the fibula, 7 *fen* to 1.2 *cun* perpendicularly.

GB 40 (*Chiuhsu, Quixu*): In the depression on the anterior inferior aspect of the lateral malleolus, 3 to 5 *fen* perpendicularly.

GB 41 (*Linchi, Linqi*): Between the fourth and the fifth metacarpal bones, 1.5 *cun* behind *Hsiahsi*, 5 *fen* to 1 *cun* perpendicularly.

GB 44 (*Chiaoyin, Foot-Qiaoyin*): About 1 *fen* below the lateral base of the fourth toe, obliquely to a depth of 1 to 2 *fen*.

Meridian Li (Liver, Tsu Chueh Yin Kan Ching, Foot–Jueyin, L)

There are 14 acupuncture points on Meridian Li (Figures 2–13 and 2–14). The 6 most frequently used are:

Li 1 (*Tatun, Dadun*): On the lateral aspect of the distal phalange of the first toe, posterior to the base of the nail, obliquely to a depth of 1 to 2 *fen*.

Li 2 (*Hsingchien, Xingjian*): About 5 *fen* behind the web of the first toe and the second toe, in front of the first and second joints of the digitorum pedis, 5 *fen* to 1 *cun* perpendicularly.

Li 3 (*Taichung, Taichong*): In the depression, in between the first and second metatarsal bones, Li 3 is 1.5 *cun* above Li 2, 5 *fen* to 1 *cun* perpendicularly.

Li 4 (*Chungfeng, Zhongfeng*): 1 *cun* anteriorly from the medial malleolus between the tendons of the extensor hallucis longus muscle and the tibialis anterior muscle, 3 to 5 *fen* perpendicularly.

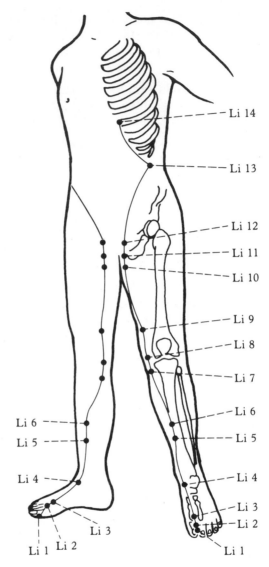

Figure 2-13.   Meridian Li (Liver, *Tsu Chueh Yin Kan Ching*, Foot–Jueyin, L)

Li 8   (*Chuchuan, Ququan*): At the medial end of the knee crease, in front of the semimembranosus muscle behind the lower end of the femur, 5 *fen* to 1.2 *cun* perpendicularly.

Li 14 (*Chimen, Qimen*): In men, the space between the sixth and the seventh ribs below the nipples; in women, Li 14 is in the space between the sixth and seventh ribs below the nipples, obliquely to a depth of 3 *fen*.

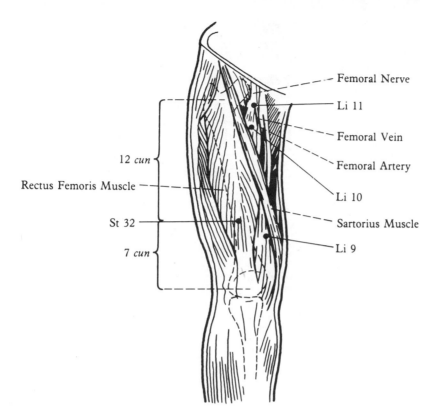

Figure 2–14. Some points on the anterior thigh in relation to other structures

Meridian Sx (Sex, Jen Mo, Ren Mo, Front Midline, Conception Vessel, M)

There are 24 acupuncture points on Meridian Sx (Figures 2–15 and 2–16). The 11 most frequently used are:

Sx 3   (*Chungchi, Zhongji*): 4 cun below the umbilicus on the midline of the abdomen, 5 *fen* to 1 *cun* perpendicularly.

Sx 6   (*Chihai, Qihai*): 1.5 cun below the umbilicus, 4 *fen* to 1 *cun* perpendicularly.

Sx 7   (*Yinjiao*): 1 cun below the umbilicus, perpendicularly, 5 *fen* to 1 *cun.*

Sx 9   (*Shuifen*): 1 cun above the umbilicus, perpendicularly, 5 *fen* to 1 *cun.*

Sx 10   (*Hsiawan, Xiawan*): 2 cun above the umbilicus, 8 *fen* to 1 *cun* perpendicularly.

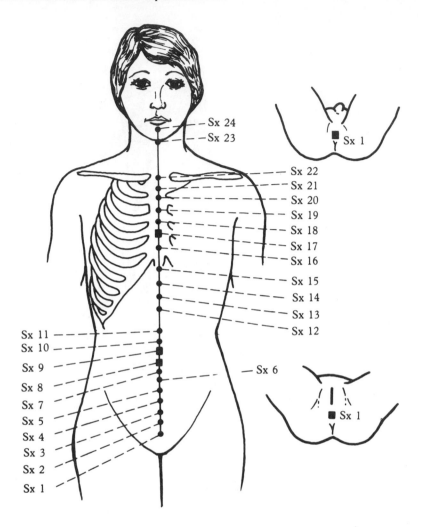

■ Forbidden Point

Figure 2–15. Meridian Sx (Sex, *Jen Mo, Ren Mo,* Front Midline, Conception Vessel, M)

Sx 12   (*Chungwan, Zhongwan*): 4 cun above the umbilicus or between the umbilicus and the costophrenic angle, 8 *fen* to 1 *cun* perpendicularly.

Sx 13   (*Shangwan*): 5 *cun* above the umbilicus, 5 *fen* to 1 *cun* perpendicularly.

Sx 17   (*Shangchung, Shanzhong*): In men, on the median line of the sternum between the two nipples; in women, on the median

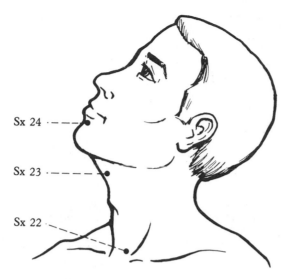

Sx 24

Sx 23

Sx 22

Figure 2–16. Sex meridian points on the face and neck

line of the sternum between the fourth and the fifth ribs, superficially downward to a depth of 3 to 5 *fen*.

Sx 22 (*Tientu, Tiantu*): In the center of the depression above the
suprasternal notch, the needle being inserted downward
alongside the trachea, obliquely downward to a depth of 5 to 7
fen, being very careful to avoid blood vessels and other vital
structures.

Sx 23 (*Lienchuan, Lianguan*): In the center of the upper border of the
hyoid bone above the laryngeal prominence, to a depth of 5 *fen*
to 1 *cun* toward the root of the tongue, being very careful to
avoid blood vessels.

Sx 24 (*Chengchiang, Chengjiang*): In the middle of the mentolabial
sulcus, upward and obliquely to a depth of 2 to 3 *fen*.

Meridian Br (Brain, Tu Mo, Du Mo, Back Midline, Governor Vessel, N)

There are 28 points on Meridian Br (Figure 2–17). The 11 most
frequently used are:

Br 1 (*Changchiang*): In between the tip of the coccyx and the anus,
2 to 5 *fen* perpendicularly.

Br 2 (*Yaoshu*): In the center of the sacral depression above the
coccyx, 4 to 6 *fen* perpendicularly.

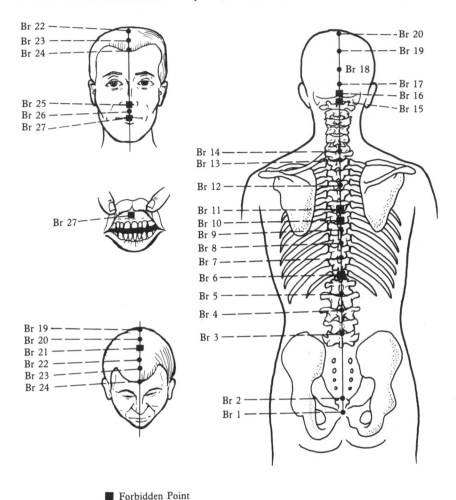

■ Forbidden Point

Figure 2-17.   Meridian Br (Brain, *Tu Mo*, *Du Mo*, Back Midline, Governor Vessel, N)

Br 3   (*Yaoyangguan*): Below the spinous process of the fourth lumbar vertebra, 3 *fen* to 1 *cun* perpendicularly.

Br 4   (*Mingmen*): Below the spinous process of the second lumbar vertebra Br 4 faces the median line of the umbilicus 5 to 8 *fen* perpendicularly.

Br 12 (*Shenchu*): Below the spinous process of the third thoracic vertebra, 3 to 5 *fen* perpendicularly.

Br 13 (*Taotao, Taodao*): Below the spinous process of the first thoracic vertebra, 5 to 8 *fen* perpendicularly.

Br 14   (*Tachui, Dazhui*): Between the spinous process of the seventh cervical vertebra and of the first thoracic vertebra, 5 to 8 *fen* perpendicularly.

Br 15   (*Yomen, Yamen*): (Forbidden) In the midline of the back of the neck 5 *fen* into the natural hairline, between the first and the second cervical vertebra, superficially 2 to 5 *fen*.

Br 16   (*Fengfu*): In the midline of the back of the neck, 1 *cun* above the natural hairline at the back of the head, in the depression below the occipital protuberance, 3 to 5 *fen* perpendicularly.

Br 20   (*Paihui, Baihui*): At the middle of the occipital scalp, 2 to 3 *fen* perpendicularly.

Br 26   (*Shanghsing, Shangxing*): Just above the middle of the philtrum of the upper lip, upward obliquely to a depth of 3 to 5 *fen*.

GENERAL REFERENCES FOR CHAPTER   2

Academy of Traditional Chinese Medicine. *An Outline of Chinese Acupuncture*. Peking: Foreign Language Press, 1975.

Anonymous. *An Explanatory Book of the Newest Illustrations of Acupuncture Points*. Hong Kong: Medicine and Health Publishing Company, 1974.

Anonymous. *An Outline of Chinese Acupuncture* (In Chinese). Peking: People's Hygiene Press, 1972.

Chang, Kui–Sun. *Anthology on Acupuncture* (In Chinese). Lanchow City, China: Gansu People's Publishing Co., 1978.

Cheong, W. C.: and Yang, C.P. *Synopsis of Chinese Acupuncture*. Hong Kong: The Light Publishing Co., 1974.

Kao, Wu. *Finest Writings on Acupuncture* (In Chinese). Shanghi: Technical Scientific Publishing Company, 1978.

Mann, Felix. *Acupuncture, The Ancient Chinese Art of Healing and How It Works Scientifically*. Vintage Books, 1973.

———. *Atlas of Acupuncture*. London: William Heinemann Medical Books, Ltd., 1973.

Shanghi College of Traditional Chinese Medicine. *Acupuncture and Moxibustion Textbook* (In Chinese). Peking: People's Health Publishing Company, 1974.

Silverstein, Martin E.: Chang, I–Lok; and Mason, Nathaniel (translators). *Acupuncture and Moxibustion, A Handbook for the Barefoot Doctors of China*. New York: Schocken Books, 1975.

Traditional Chinese Medical Institute. *A Concise Acupuncture Textbook* (In Chinese). Peking: People's Medical Publisher, 1978.

chapter 3

SPECIAL ACUPUNCTURE POINTS

Besides the acupuncture points on the fourteen classical meridians, some other useful points have been discovered and designated as Extraordinary Points (Ex). Some acupuncture texts diagram these as being on special meridians which intersect with the major meridians. These are usually classified in accordance with the part of the body on which they are located. Non-meridian acupuncture points and areas which affect specific parts of the body have been discovered on the ears, soles of the feet, and face. Some of these are especially useful for acupuncture analgesia.

EXTRAORDINARY POINTS ON THE HEAD AND NECK

Ex 1 (*Yingtang*): Midway between the eyebrows, barely 3 *fen* beneath the skin. This point is considered useful for relieving nasal congestion, headache, and dizziness.

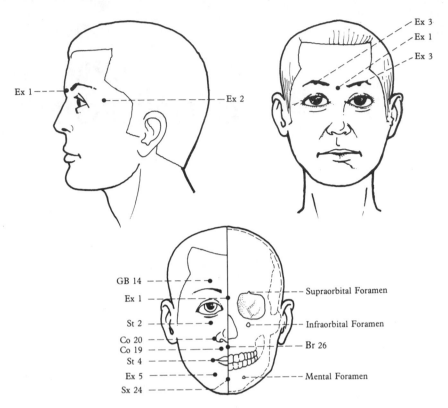

Figure 3–1. Extraordinary points on the head

Ex 2　(*Taiyang*): In the shallow depression 1 *cun* posterior to the midpoint between the lateral limit of the eyebrow and the outer canthus of the eye. It is used for treating migraine, tic doulour-eux, and facial paralysis.

Ex 3　(*Yuyao*): Between the eyebrows, 3 to 5 *fen* obliquely upward. It is used for relieving forehead pain, eye diseases, and facial paralysis.

Ex 4　(*Qiuhou*): On the cheek under the eye on the level of St 1, between St 1 and the external canthus of the eye, perpendicu-larly, 3 to 5 *fen*. This point is too close to the eye to be safe for beginners, but it has been found useful for treating myopia, atrophy of the optic nerve, optic neuritis, glaucoma, and tur-bidity of the vitreous humor.

Ex 5　(*Jiachengjiang*): 1 *cun* lateral to Sx 24, perpendicularly 2 to 3 *fen*. This point is used for treating trigeminal neuralgia and facial paralysis.

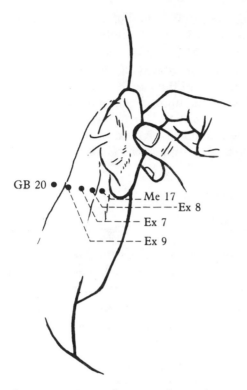

Figure 3–2. Extraordinary points in relation to classical points

Ex 6   (*Sishencong*): 1 *cun* posterior, anterior, and lateral to Br 20, 2 to 5 *fen* obliquely laterally. This point is used for treating headache, dizziness, and epilepsy.

Ex 7   (*Yiming*): 1 *cun* posterior to Me 17 on the lower border of the mastoid, 2 to 5 *fen* perpendicularly. It is used for treating atrophy of the optic nerve, myopia, cataracts, tinnitus, insomnia, and parotitis. (See Figure 3–2.)

Ex 8   (*Anmian I*): Between Me 17 and Ex 7, perpendicularly 2 to 5 *fen*. It is used for treating insomnia and schizophrenia.

Ex 9   (*Anmian II*): Between Ex 7 and GB 20, perpendicularly, 3 to 6 *fen*. It is used for treating insomnia.

Ex 10   (*Jinjin, Yuye*): This point is under the tongue and is too dangerous for use in the United States.

Ex 11   (*Zengyin*): In a depression just lateral to the thyroid cartilage, 3 to 5 *fen* upward and medially. It is used for treating speech disorders.

Ex 12   (*Shanglianquan*): 1 *cun* below the midpoint of the mandible in midline, 3 to 8 *fen* obliquely upward. It is used for treating speech disorders.

Ex 13   (*Jingbi*): 3 *cun* lateral of the sternoclavicular notch on the upper border of the clavicle, 2 to 3 *fen* obliquely upward. It is too close to the apex of the lung and large blood vessels of the neck to be safe for beginners, but it is sometimes used for treating numbness or pain of the arm and hand or to relieve paralysis of the upper extremity.

EXTRAORDINARY POINTS OF THE THORAX, ABDOMEN, AND PELVIS

Ex 14   (*Weishang*): 2 *cun* above the umbilicus, 4 *cun* lateral to the midline, 3 to 8 *fen* obliquely toward the umbilicus. It is used for treating weakness of abdominal muscles.

Ex 15   (*Weibao*): On a level with Sx 4 in the inguinal groove about 4 *cun* lateral to Sx 4, obliquely 3 to 5 *fen* downward. It is used to treat weakness of pelvic muscles.

Ex 16   (*Abdomen–Zigong*): 3 *cun* lateral to Sx 3, perpendicularly, 3 to 5 *fen*. It is used for treating dyspareunia and constipation.

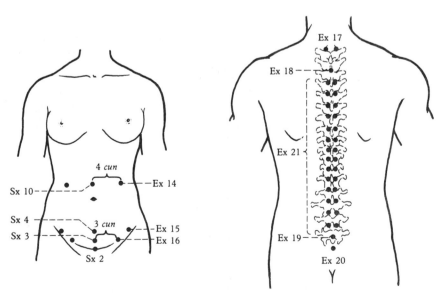

Figure 3–3.   Extraordinary points on the torso

Ex 17   (*Dingchuan*): 0.5 (5 *fen*) *cun* lateral to Br 14, obliquely medially, 2 to 5 *fen*. It is used for treating bronchial asthma and chronic bronchitis.

Ex 18   (*Wuming*): In the depression below the spinous process of the second thoracic vertebra, 2 to 5 *fen* obliquely upward. It is used for hyperactivity.

Ex 19   (*Shiqizhui*): In the depression below the spinous process of the fifth lumbar vertebra, perpendicularly, 3 to 8 *fen*. It is used for relief of lumbosacral pain and stiffness.

Ex 20   (*Yaoqi*): 2 *cun* above the coccyx, obliquely upward 5 to 8 *fen*. It is used for treating epilepsy.

Ex 21   (*Huatuojiaji*): A series of points about 5 *fen* lateral to the midline and about 5 *fen* apart from the neck to the sacrum, 3 to 5 *fen* obliquely medially. These points are used mostly for treating pain in their areas.

EXTRAORDINARY POINTS OF THE
UPPER EXTREMITY

Ex 22   (*Jianzhong*): In the middle of the deltoid muscle midway between Co 15 and Co 14, perpendicularly 5 *fen* to 1 *cun*. It is used for treating paralysis of the upper extremity.

Ex 23   (*Bizhong*): At the midpoint of an imaginary line between the cubital transverse crease and the transverse crease of the wrist, on the midline of the medial aspect of the forearm, perpendicularly 5 *fen* to 1 *cun*. It is used for treating chest pain and paralysis of the arms.

Ex 24   (*Erbai*): 4 points of ambiguous location on the forearm, used for treating hemorrhoids. Since good surgical treatment for hemorrhoids is readily available in the United States, there is not much point in using these points here. (See Figure 3–4.)

Ex 25   (*Zhongquan*): On the wrist in a depression on the radial aspect of the tendon of the extensor digitorum communis muscle, perpendicularly 2 to 5 *fen*. It is used to relieve dyspnea and wrist disorders. (See Figure 3–5).

Ex 26   (*Luozhen*): On the back of the hand between the second and third metacarpal bones, 5 *fen* proximal to the metacarpo–phalangeal joints, 2 to 4 *fen* obliquely laterally.

Ex 27   (*Yatong*): On the back of the hand between the third and fourth metacarpal bones 5 *fen* proximal to the metacarpo–phalangeal

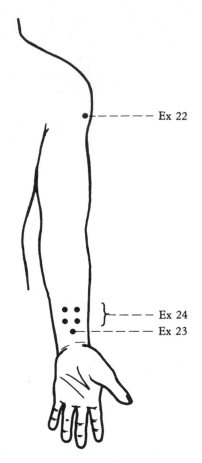

Figure 3–4.   Extraordinary points 22, 23, and 24

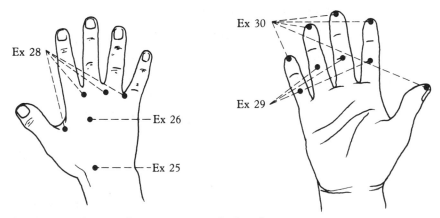

Figure 3–5.   Extraordinary points on the hands

joints, 2 to 4 *fen* perpendicularly. It is used for treating stiffness of the neck and torticollis.

Ex 28   (*Baxie*): On the back of the webs between each of the fingers, 8 points in all, 2 to 5 *fen* obliquely proximally. These points are used to treat disorders of the finger joints, numbness of the fingers, headache, and pain in the neck.

Ex 29   (*Sifeng*): On the palmar surface in the transverse creases of the proximal interphalangeal joints of the four fingers (not the thumbs) of the hands, 8 points in all, 1 to 2 *fen* perpendicularly. These points are used for treating anorexia and chronic coughs.

Ex 30   (*Shixuan*): 10 points on the tips of the fingers, including the thumbs, 2 to 4 *fen*. These points are used to treat shock, coma, and heat stroke.

EXTRAORDINARY POINTS ON THE LOWER EXTREMITY

See Figures 3–6 and 3–7.

Ex 31   (*Heding*): On the midpoint of the upper border of the patella, perpendicularly 3 to 5 *fen*. This point is used to treat pain and stiffness of the knee joint.

Ex 32   (*Xiyan*): At the lower margins of the patella, both medially and laterally, perpendicularly 5 *fen* to 1 *cun*. These 4 points are used to treat disorders of the knee joints.

Ex 33   (*Lanwei*): 2 *cun* below St 36, points where tenderness may appear to facilitate diagnosis of appendicitis, perpendicularly 5 *fen* to 1 *cun*. This point is used to treat paralysis and paresis of the lower extremity.

Ex 34   (*Linghou*): Just posterior and inferior to the head of the fibula, perpendicularly 2 to 4 *fen*. This point is used to treat sciatica and paralysis of the lower extremity.

Ex 35   (*Dannang*): 1 *cun* below GB 34 where tenderness is experienced by the patient perpendicularly 3 to 8 *fen*. It is used to treat paralysis of the lower extremities.

Ex 36   (*Bafeng*): On the back of the foot, altogether 8 points just proximal to the webs between each of the toes, 3 to 10 *fen* obliquely and proximally. These points are used to treat numbness and pain of the toes and dorsum of the foot.

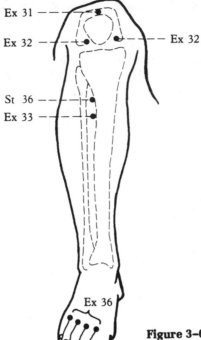

Ex 31

Ex 32 — — Ex 32

St 36

Ex 33

Ex 36

Figure 3–6.   Extraordinary points on the front of the leg and foot

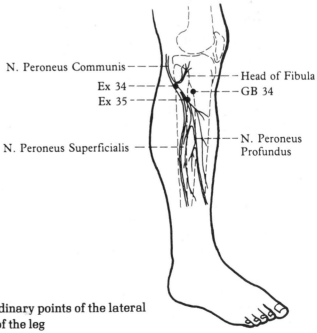

N. Peroneus Communis

Ex 34 — Head of Fibula

Ex 35 — GB 34

N. Peroneus Superficialis — N. Peroneus Profundus

Figure 3–7.   Extraordinary points of the lateral aspect of the leg

AURICULAR POINTS: ACUPUNCTURE POINTS AND AREAS ON THE EAR

The practice of auriculotherapy is based on the concept that there are parts of the ear which can be related to specific parts of the rest of the body for acupuncture treatment. The general location of these points or areas of the ear is determined by viewing the ear as a diagram of a near–term fetus in the uterus with the head down at the lobe of the ear, the back along the outer margin of the ear, and the abdomen, arms, and legs proximal toward the ear's attachment to the head. The location of these specific points and areas on the ear can be learned much more easily by studying diagrams (Figure 3–8) and manikins than from anatomical descriptions of them.

There is considerable variation of opinion among the authors of acupuncture textbooks as well as practicing acupuncturists, on the location of the points and areas on the ears. Those presented here are a composite of auricular point diagrams in many acupuncture textbooks.

Ear points have been mapped for treating pain and ailments in every part of the body. They have also been used for obesity and addiction to drugs, alcohol, and tobacco. Acupuncture points on the ears are especially useful for surgical analgesia of most parts of the body because they enable the acupuncturist to avoid placing needles near the surgical field. These points are useful for the emergency relief of pain from accidental physical injuries, particularly when it is unwise to move the patient. Paramedical emergency personnel, if trained in these techniques, could supply this type of relief. The use of ear points does not require the removal of clothing and is therefore more acceptable than classical acupuncture to many people who are in severe pain or who are extremely modest.

Some Americans have popularized the practice of inserting a surgical staple through the upper cartilaginous part of the ear for treatment of addictions and obesity. These staples are sometimes left in place for months. This technique is less effective and more dangerous than regular acupuncture treatment. The staple becomes a source of infection and may cause sloughing of ear tissue or keloid formation. A variation of this technique is the insertion of very small needles in the ear leaving them in place for many days or weeks. These needles frequently fall out. They may become lodged in the external ear canal, causing irritation, infection, and pain; or they may even migrate to and damage the eardrum. The author does not recommend either of these practices.

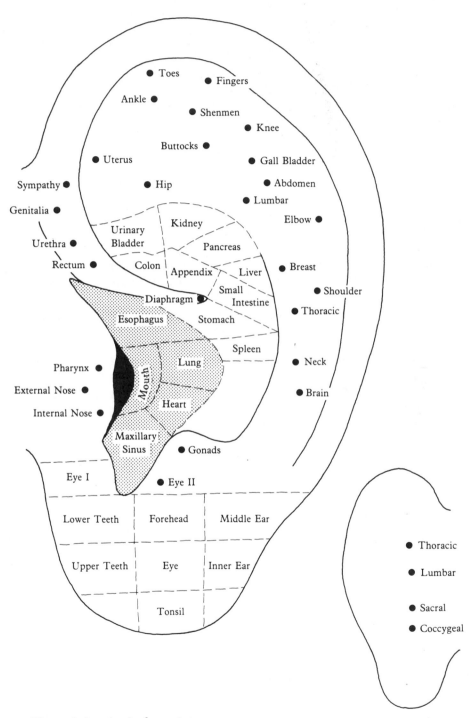

Figure 3–8.   Auricular points

ACUPUNCTURE POINTS AND AREAS
ON THE SOLES OF THE FEET

Points and areas on the soles of the feet have been found useful for anesthetizing or treating various parts of the head, neck, abdomen, and pelvis. The location of these points and areas has been determined empirically by acupuncturists in China and elsewhere who were trying to find points for surgical analgesia. They sought points which were as remote as possible from the surgical field. These points are also useful for providing emergency relief of pain to injured patients without moving them or removing their clothes. There is some variation of opinion about the precise location of these points and about the size and shape of the areas diagrammed in different acupuncture text-books.

There seems to be general agreement that points for the scalp and pituitary gland are on the big toe. Points for the eyes are on the second and middle toes, while points for the ears are on the fourth and little toes. Points and areas for the neck and torso are located proximally. Areas for hemorrhoid analgesia are located around the edges of the heels. As with points and areas on the ears, it is easier to learn the location of these points by studying diagrams than from anatomical descriptions of them. (See Figure 3–9).

In order to determine precisely where to insert the needles for an individual patient for a specific surgical procedure, the acupuncturist should test the relative effectiveness of possible sites the day before the surgery and mark the ones he chooses to use.

FACIAL POINTS FOR ANALGESIA

Although there are classical and extraordinary points on the face, there are also special points for analgesia of certain parts of the body. These are recently discovered points, and there is still considerable controversy about their precise location. (See Figure 3–10).

PRIVATE ACUPUNCTURE POINTS

Traditional acupuncturists who have been taught by old masters, or who come from families of acupuncturists, will usually have some favorite points discovered by their teachers or ancestors. These points are regarded as secret.

Any acupuncturist who has practiced this art for many years is likely to have a few points that he has discovered experimentally on his

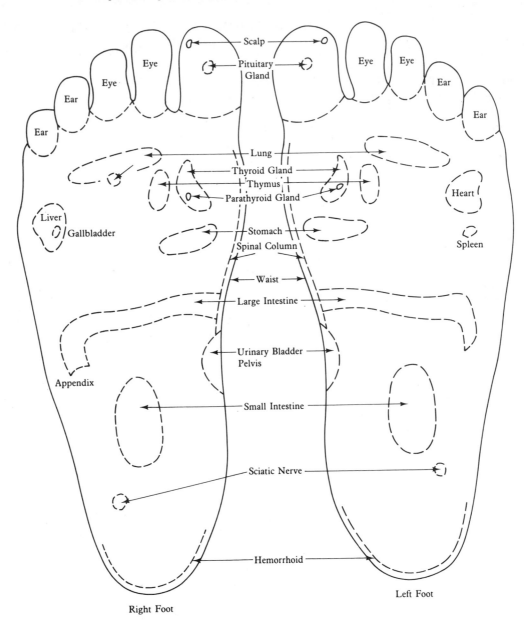

Figure 3–9.   Acupuncture points and areas on the soles of the feet

own. Although acupuncture has been practiced for thousands of years, it is still considered to be in a process of evolution. The goal is to find points which will be effective enough so that as few points as possible need to be used to produce surgical analgesia or to give effective treatment.

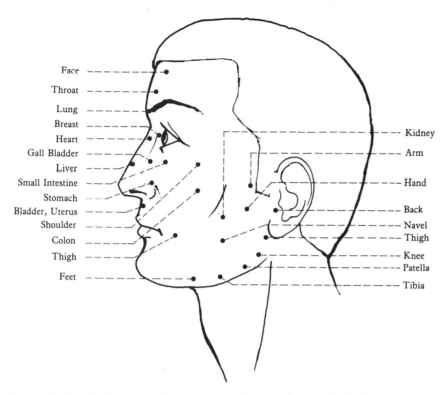

Figure 3–10.   Facial points for analgesia of some parts of the body

GENERAL REFERENCES FOR CHAPTER   3

Academy of Traditional Chinese Medicine. *An Outline of Chinese Acupuncture.* pp. 204–216, 269–280 Peking: Foreign Language Press, 1975.

Anonymous. *An Explanatory Book of the Newest Illustrations of Acupuncture Points.* 44–89. Hong Kong: Medicine and Health Publishing Company, 1974.

Cheong, S. C.: and Yang, C.P. *Synopsis of Chinese Acupuncture.* pp. 84–97. Hong Kong: The Light Publishing Company, 1974.

Nogier, P.F.M. *Treatise of Auriculo–Therapy.* France: Maisonneuve, 1972.

chapter 4

ACUPUNCTURE THEORY

The meridian system may be thought of as a radio network in which the acupuncture points are transmitters and the vital organs, receivers. The meridians are the invisible, intangible lines along which messages are sent from the acupuncture points to various parts of the body. The messages sent by insertion of needles into the acupuncture points are either to increase or decrease activity, to become more sensitive or less sensitive, depending on how and where the needles are inserted. The ancient Chinese discovered that needles inserted into some acupuncture points stimulated while needles in other acupuncture points sedated. They also observed that, in some points, the way in which the needle was inserted determined whether its effect would be sedation or stimulation.

INTERNAL COMMUNICATION

Before the invention of wireless radio transmission, it was difficult for people to believe that something invisible and intangible could have scientific reality. Now that we use radio and television regularly, however, it should no longer be incomprehensible that the human body could have a fiberless communication system as well as a system in which the nerve fibers may be compared with telephone wires. We should be able to consider the possibility that our bodies have a radio–like network as well as a telephone–like network plus the other systems which cooperate with each other to sustain life. When one organ or body system becomes overactive or underactive, it upsets the functioning of other parts of the body because the various parts of the body are interdependent and must all work together harmoniously if good health is to be maintained.

Each part of the body has its own characteristic way of warning us when something is wrong. Pain, increased temperature, swelling, vomiting, bleeding, constipation, fatigue, depression, weakness, paralysis, and paresthesia are some of the warnings which we recognize as symptoms of disease. The acupuncturists see all these symptoms as indications that the energy–transmission (radio control) system of the body is malfunctioning. They attempt to correct the malfunction by inserting needles in the manner they consider appropriate into the points (transmitting stations) which they expect will send a message of stimulation or sedation to the organ or system causing the malfunction responsible for the undesirable symptoms.

A well–balanced, smoothly–operating internal radio transmission system maintains the body in such good health that it is resistant to invasion from noxious factors in the external environment such as bacteria, excessive cold, heat, or humidity. It also promotes the rapid healing of wounds and retards the process of decay or aging.

PSYCHOSOMATIC CONSIDERATIONS

There are many ancient Chinese proverbs about how to behave or what attitude to take toward various life situations. There is a meridian with a name which can be translated as "Brain Meridian." Nevertheless, the ancient Chinese did not develop many theories specifically about how one's own thoughts and emotions can affect the functioning of various parts of his body. Until Mao's "Little Red Book" related ideology to health, there were no readily recognizable Chinese theories of psychosomatic medicine. Our own theories of psychosomatic medicine, however, fit in very well with Chinese meridian theory.

Our sense organs can be considered receptors of stimuli from the external environment which transmit the messages they receive to our brains and the meridian system. The brain's function is to sort, store, and send messages it receives. The ancient Chinese believed that all parts of the body could communicate with all other parts via the meridian system and thereby influence the function and symptoms of other parts. According to this theory, it would therefore be possible for emotions produced by the brain in response to external or internal stimuli to be responsible for disturbing the function of any part of the body. Instead of attempting to relieve psychogenic disturbances with psychotropic drugs, acupuncturists attempt to rectify the situation by inserting their needles into the acupuncture points to correct the imbalance of *Yin–Yang* (negative–positive energy) in the disturbed area. In this sense acupuncture employs physics rather than chemistry to treat malfunctions with the expectation that energy changes will lead to the desired biochemical changes.

It is possible to classify human emotions as either *Yin, Yang* or a combination of both. Anger is a *Yang* emotion of which fear and hatred are *Yin* counterparts. If we convert fear or hatred to anger, we feel more energetic and are likely to take action against the object of our distress. If we suppress anger, we feel hatred and fear which dissipate our vital energy and cause various parts of our bodies to malfunction. Joy is a *Yang* emotion of which apathy is the *Yin* counterpart. If we express our joy with song, dance, or making love, we get a general feeling of well–being unless we continue the joy–inspired behavior so long that we become tired. Then we relax and sleep or become apathetic. A person whose life situation is pleasant, comfortable, and free from anxiety, is likely to become lazy, soft, and sluggish unless he expresses joy about such a situation in a creative manner. He must maintain a balance between the *Yin* and *Yang* aspects of his emotions and behavior.

In considering the psychosomatic theory that arthritis is aggravated, perhaps even caused, by repressed anger or hostility, we could speculate that excessive *Yang* accumulates around joints and causes the malfunction and eventual deformity. Then we could say that acupuncture sends messages of sedation to these areas which restore the *Yin–Yang* balance and promote relief of symptoms. Our psychosomatic theories, however, are probably not adequate to explain all the effects of acupuncture in arthritis or other ailments.

BASIC CONCEPTS OF TRADITIONAL CHINESE MEDICINE [1,2]

Although it is possible to learn acupuncture without understanding or accepting Chinese medical theories, it may facilitate selection of points and techniques to be familiar with some of the concepts referred to in Chinese medical literature. There may seem to be discrepancies in the classification of some organs according to these concepts. For instance, the lung is considered *Piao* (external) but also *Tsang* (internal). Some of these ancient Chinese concepts related to acupuncture therapy are as follows:

Yin and Yang

Satisfactory definitions of *Yin* and *Yang* are lacking, but one may classify *Yin* and *Yang* as two different types of energy. *Yin* is associated with preservation and storage of internal energy; *Yang* is associated with the utilization of energy. A "*Yin* condition" is a deficiency disease or chronic disorder with insidious development. Weakness, muscle wasting, pallor, and depression are the most common symptoms. A "*Yang* condition" is a disease with acute onset and obvious development. The most common symptoms are fever and restlessness. Different combinations of acupuncture points are chosen for treating patients with the same ailment but different *Yin* and *Yang* symptoms. In the United States, most people treated by acupuncture are considered to have *Yin* conditions.

Piao (Biao, Surface, External) and Li (Internal)

Structures which are in contact with the external environment are classified as *Piao*; for example, the skin, digestive and respiratory tracts. Other internal structures and visceral organs are classified as *Li*. These concepts are used to locate the origin of illness and the translocations of symptoms and toxicity produced by malfunctions of organs. In a general way, *Piao* is related to *Yang*, and *Li* is related to *Yin*.

Shiu (Emptiness) and Shih, (Fullness)

Shiu indicates that internal energy has been severely depleted while the disease process is still active. The pulses of the patient are usually very weak and thready, while abdominal muscles show little tone or strength. These symptoms indicate a deficiency of energy. In such cases acupuncture therapy should be moderate and cautious. This concept is somewhat similar to *Yin* and *Li*. On the other hand, if the body seems to have resistance and is fighting against the disease and the pulses are strong and the abdominal muscles firm, the patient's condition is described as *Shih*, somewhat similar to *Yang* and *Piao*.

These concepts are useful in determining which acupuncture points and which needle techniques should be used for patients in different physiological and psychological states. In general, Chinese acupuncture is thought to exert its therapeutic effects by stimulating the intrinsic normal body functions to restore homeostasis and natural body resistance to external infectious agents, such as bacteria and viruses, as well as by stimulating metabolism and relieving tension.

Tsang and Fu

Classical Chinese medical books divide the visceral structures into two groups: *Tsang* (heart, liver, spleen, lung, kidney, and vascular) and *Fu* (small intestine, gall bladder, stomach, colon, urinary bladder, and metabolism). The six *Tsang* structures are thought to maintain the supply of internal energy and homeostasis. The six *Fu* structures are mainly digestive and excretory in nature and in contact with the external environment. Most of the *Fu* structures are therefore classified as *Piao* (external) and the *Tsang* as *Li* (internal). *Tsang* is related to *Yin* and *Fu* is related to *Yang*. There is one meridian for each of the *Tsang* and *Fu* organs or systems.

Han (Cold) and Reh (Hot)

Han is a concept used to describe an afebrile illness and is related to *Yin*. *Reh* is used to describe a patient with a fever and is related to *Yang*.

Ching-Lo (Meridians)

The fundamental concept of the body energy system has meridian lines of energy flow (*Ching–Lo*) connecting all tissues and organs of the body in functional integrity. *Ching* meridian lines run mostly vertically. *Lo* lines run horizontally and represent branches or connecting anastomoses of the vertical (*Ching*) lines.

There are twelve paired meridians, one meridian which travels along the midline of the back (*Du Mai, Tu Mo,* Governing Vessel, or Brain Meridian), and one meridian which travels along the ventral midline (*Ren Mai, Jen Mo,* Conception vessel, or Sex Meridian). Most of the Classical Chinese acupuncture points (*Loci*) belong to these 14 major meridians, as described in Chapter 2.

Sequence of Energy Flow

Without knowledge of modern neuroanatomy and physiology, ancient Chinese physicians utilized cutaneous stimulation empirically to treat visceral disorders based on the experiences passed down by their ancestors. Usually a needle was inserted into the extremities to treat the pain syndrome of a remote region or malfunction of some visceral organ. To explain the effectiveness of acupuncture, classical Chinese medical books describe the circulation of energy in the body.[3] They say that energy flows along the twelve paired meridians in the order indicated in the following schematic diagram (Figure 4–1) and that acupuncturists can increase or decrease the energy of a meridian by stimulating or sedating the meridian immediately preceding it according to the direction of energy flow.

Recent attempts have been made to trace meridian channels and energy flow by scientific methods. A Leningrad surgeon, Mikhail Kizmich Gaikin, using the techniques of photography in a high–frequency electrical field (originally discovered by Semyon and Valentina Kirlian), has found that the places of greatest bioluminescence on the human body correspond with the Chinese acupuncture points.[4] This observation led to development of the tobiscope, an instrument which improves the accuracy of acupuncture needle placement. Research on high–frequency photography is now being performed at the Kazakh State University in Al–ata, Russia, and also at several universities in

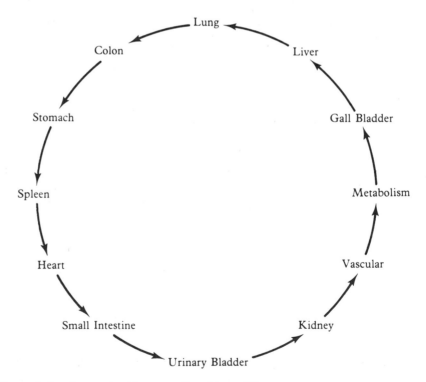

Figure 4–1.   Sequence of energy flow in meridians

the United States. Gaikin's discovery led to the proposition that the high–frequency photographic image actually depicts the energy flow along the meridians and acupuncture points of the human body.

Concept and Law of the Five Essences[5]

The ancient Chinese believed that there are five basic essences which interact in a creative cycle to produce all forms of matter. These essences are Fire, Water, Earth, Wood, and Air. An old Chinese translation for this last essence is "something of great value," which has been translated as "gold" and later as "metal." "Air" seems a better translation of this essence from the standpoint of the original meaning as well as the symbolism involved in this concept. Each essence has a relative proportion of *Yin* and *Yang* energy manifested in a set of characteristics. According to Chinese theories, the basis of the five essences is the antagonism and the reaction of *Yin* and *Yang*. Scientific explanations of the *Yin* and *Yang* concept and the five essences are in the process of research and development.[6]

According to Chinese theory, the vital organs in the human body are characterized by different manifestations of *Yin* and *Yang* energy. Each of the paired meridians is named after an organ or system with which it is considered to be closely associated. These meridians are classified as related to one of the five essences and basically *Yin* or *Yang* as follows:

Heart and Vascular—*Yin*
Small Intestine and Metabolism—*Yang* } Fire

Spleen—*Yin*
Stomach—*Yang* } Earth

Lungs—*Yin*
Colon—*Yang* } Air

Kidney—*Yin*
Urinary Bladder—*Yang* } Water

Liver—*Yin*
Gall Bladder—*Yang* } Wood

In the creative–destructive cycle of the five essences, the visceral organs and related functions are thought to enhance and to hinder one another. The theory of the five essences was developed to explain the interactions of the internal organs and body systems. (Figure 4–2). The name of the visceral organ in Chinese often implies its functions and related structures. For example, the Chinese name

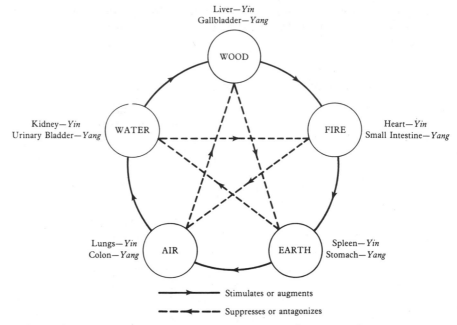

Figure 4-2.   Relationships of the five essences and associated viscera

for lungs (*fei*) implies respiration, its effects on the body and skin, the energy generated by oxidation, and also catabolism.

The five essences concept is also used to describe a person's physical appearance, personality, and psychic energy. For example, someone with a florid complexion who sweats excessively and has a quick temper is thought to be dominated by the essence Fire. This type of person is considered likely to develop ailments of the heart, the *Yin* organ of this essence. The five essence theory follows the creative and destructive interactions of the essences in nature. Accordingly, the *first law of acupuncture*, also called "the law of the five essences," is: Acupuncturists should not ignore simultaneously stimulatory and inhibitory effects of the treatment on different organs. For example, when the heart meridian is stimulated, the energy of the spleen meridian will be increased; the energy of the liver meridian, however, will be reduced.

Pulse Diagnosis and the Reciprocal Law of Acupuncture

The *reciprocal law of acupuncture* is that meridians represented by the left wrist pulses dominate those represented by the right wrist pulses; conversely, the right ones may hinder the left ones in stimulating energy and blood circulation during acupuncture therapy. The possibility that right wrist pulses are dominant in left–handed people, however, should be considered.

Evaluating pulses has been developed as a diagnostic procedure by traditional Chinese acupuncturists. They believe that there are three pairs of pulses on each wrist: (1) *Tsun*, between the transverse stria of the wrist and styloid protuberance; (2) *Kuan*, at the level of the styloid protuberance; and (3) *Chih*, above the styloid protuberance. At each position, there are said to be two pulses: a superficial *Yang* pulse and a deep *Yin* pulse. The left wrist is considered *Yang* and the right wrist is considered *Yin*. Some acupuncturists now use electronic pulse detectors to identify these. The frequency and amplitude of different pulses can be registered by pen–recorders.

The twelve pulse readings are considered indicative of the energy conditions and the activities of the twelve meridians and organs. A bounding pulse is thought to indicate an excess of energy. Chinese acupuncturists say there are 23 different types of pulses characterized by frequency and amplitude differences. The meridians and organs represented by the pulses at the same position on both wrists are thought to obey the law that the left wrist meridian dominates the right one. For example, the deep pulse at the left *Tsun* position indicates the activity of the heart meridian which dominates the lung meridian which is represented by the deep pulse on the right wrist at the same position. Acupuncture stimulation applied to the heart meridian will affect the lung meridian simultaneously, according to this law. The traditional acupuncturist is concerned with these reciprocal interactions. Since all these "pulses" are on the radial artery, however, near the same position where Americans and Europeans usually check a patient's pulse, it seems strange and misleading to consider them as separate, and it is no longer considered necessary for an acupuncturist to learn pulse diagnosis.

The Commanding Loci of Meridians[7]

The commanding *loci* are key acupuncture points which are considered to have crucial influence on the functions of meridians and corresponding visceral organs. They can have special significance in clinical practice, and it may be useful to know their classification and names.

On the limbs, there are five commanding loci which are named according to their locations. *Tsing* (the well) points are on the tips of the fingers and toes. Like a well where underground water emerges, the *Tsing* acupuncture points are considered to be the emerging points of energy. *Yung* (radiant) points are on the branches of small streams of energy. *Yu* (assent) points on the hands and feet are considered to be the junctions of small streams of energy flow. *Ching* (passage) points above the wrist and ankle are the main passages of energy flow. *Ho* (meeting) points at the elbows and knees are the sites of convergence of energy channels. These important loci have their characteristic meanings, properties, and therapeutic effects. They are supposedly named according to energy flow. The properties of the five commanding loci are listed below:

PROPERTIES OF THE COMMANDING LOCI

Five Commanding Loci	Energy Flow	Anatomical Location	Five Essences	
			Yang Meridians	Yin Meridians
Tsing (well)	Emerging	Tips of fingers and toes	Air	Wood
Yung (radiant)	Streaming	Base of fingers and toes	Water	Fire
Yu (assent)	Filling	Hands and feet	Wood	Earth
Ching (passage)	Passing	Wrists and ankles	Fire	Air
Ho (meeting)	Meeting	Elbows and knees	Earth	Water

This chart shows that the characteristics of the commanding loci are classified according to the concept of the five essences. The interrelationships between these loci are accordingly said to be controlled by the Law of the Five Essences. The acupuncturist, therefore, may choose acupuncture points in sequential order following the direction of energy flow and creative cycles of the five essences for stimulation or tonification, and the reverse for sedation.

Origin Loci (Yuan)

The origin locus is thought to be the point where the organ transports its *Yin–Yang* energy to its meridian. For this reason, the origin locus is often used for the treatment of a diseased organ. Following is a list of the origin loci of the twelve paired meridians.

Meridians	Origin Loci
Lu (Lung, A, or I)	Lu 9 (Taiyuan)
Co (Colon, Large Intestine, B or II)	Co 4 (Hoku)

Meridians	Origin Loci
St (Stomach, Gastric, C or III)	St 42 (Chungyang)
Sp (Spleen, D, or IV)	Sp 3 (Taipei)
He (Heart, E, or V)	He 7 (Shenmen)
Si (Small Intestine, F, or VI)	SI 4 (Wanku)
UB (Urinary Bladder, G, or VII)	UB 64 (Chingku)
Ki (Kidney, Renal, H, or VIII)	Ki 6 (Taihsi)
Va (Vascular, Pericardium, I, or IX)	Va 7 (Taling)
Me (Metabolism, Triple Warmer, J, or X)	Me 4 (Yangchih)
GB (Gall Bladder, Biliary, K, or XI)	GB 40 (Chiuhsu)
Li (Liver, L, or XII)	Li 3 (Taichung)

Accumulating Loci (Hsi)

The accumulating *loci* of meridians represent the locations where energy is thought to accumulate. The accumulating *loci* are used for treating chronic and severe ailments. The accumulating *loci* of the twelve paired meridians are listed as follows:

Meridians	Accumulating Loci
Lu (Lung, A, or I)	Lu 6 (Kungtsiu)
Co (Colon, Large Intestine, B, or II)	Co 7 (Wenliu)
St (Stomach, Gastric, C, or III)	St 6 (Chiache)
Sp (Spleen, D, or IV)	Sp 8 (Tichi)
He (Heart, E, or V)	He 6 (Yinhsi)
SI (Small Intestine, F, or VI)	SI 6 (Yanglao)
UB (Urinary Bladder, G, or VII)	UB 63 (Chinmen)
Ki (Kidney, Renal, H, or VIII)	Ki 5 (Shiuchuan)
Va (Vascular, Pericardium, I, or IX)	Va 4 (Hsimen)
Me (Metabolism, Triple Warmer, J, or X)	Me 7 (Hiutsung)
GB (Gall Bladder, Biliary, K, or XI)	GB 36 (Waichiu)
Li (Liver, L, or XII)	Li 6 (Chungtu)

Anastomosis Points (Lo)

The primary functions of anastomosis points are the communications between the Yin and Yang meridians, the internal and the external visceral structures (Tsang and Fu). The distribution of the fifteen anastomosis points and the Yin–Yang energy to the fourteen meridians are listed according to their anatomical locations.

The distribution of fifteen anastomosis points of the meridians are listed below.

ANASTOMOSIS POINTS (Lo)

Arm	Anastomosis Points
Lu Meridian, Lung	Lu 7
Va Meridian, Vascular	Va 6
He Meridian, Heart	He 5
Co Meridian, Colon	Co 6
Me Meridian, Metabolism	Me 5
SI Meridian, Small Intestine	SI 7

Leg	Anastomosis Points
Sp Meridian, Spleen	Sp 4
Li Meridian, Liver	Li 4
Ki Meridian, Kidney	Ki 4
St Meridian, Stomach	St 40
GB Meridian, Gall Bladder	GB 37
UB Meridian, Urinary Bladder	UB 58

Trunk	
Br Meridian, Brain	Br 1
Sx Meridian, Sex	Sx 15
Sp Spleen anastomosis branch	Sp 21

On the thorax and the abdominal wall, there are some special acupuncture points which are located close to the visceral organs, and they are thought to have mutual influence with the *commanding loci* on the back. These acupuncture points are called *"Mo loci"* on the ventral side of the body and *"Shu loci"* on the dorsal side. To treat chronic malfunctions of the visceral organs, the *Mo loci* are often used. The *Mo loci* are characterized as *Yin* for all the organs. The *Yang loci* of the visceral organs are the *Shu loci* and are considered important gates for controlling the circulation of energy in and out of organs near them. For this reason, the *Yin locus* of the organ is used for acute and rapidly spreading disease. The *Mo loci* and *Shu loci* of the visceral organs are listed below.

THE MO AND SHU LOCI OF VISCERAL ORGANS

Visceral Organ or System	Mo Locus	Shu Locus
Lungs	Lu 1	UB 13
Vascular	Sx 17	UB 14
Heart		UB 15
Liver	Li 14	UB 18
Gall Bladder	Ki 24	UB 20
Stomach	Sx 12	UB 21
Metabolism	Sx 55	UB 22
Colon	St 25	UB 25
Kidney	Ki 25	UB 23
Small Intestine	Sx 4	UB 27
Urinary Bladder	Sx 3	UB 28

Converging (Wei) Loci

Besides the above mentioned *loci* of meridians and organs, there are eight *Wei* (converging) *loci* which are thought to control different types of tissues, visceral structures, and energy transfers. These are sometimes called the "eight influential points." Diseases related to a type of tissue in general can be treated by using its converging *loci*. They are listed on the following page.

CONVERGING LOCI

Tissue Type and Energy	Converging Loci
Tsang (Yin viscera)	Li 13
Fu (Yang viscera)	Sx 12
Chi (energy)	Sx 17
Blood	UB 17
Bone	UB 11
Bone Marrow	GB 39
Tendon–muscle	GB 34
Meridians	Lu 9

Special Points

Besides the 14 major meridians, some acupuncturists claim to have discovered six more meridians. The therapeutic value of the six special (Chih) meridians, however, is not clearly established. Together with the sex and brain meridians they are called the "eight special meridians." Points on them are the "extraordinary points" diagrammed in Chapter 3. The connecting loci (anastomosis points) between the twelve paired meridians and the eight special meridians have been designated as follows: Sp 4, Va 6, SI 3, UB 63, GB 15, Me 5, Lu 7, and Ki 3. Each of these connecting loci is thought to have simultaneous influence on its own meridian and on the special meridians to exert a widespread therapeutic effect.

There has always been considerable controversy about the deep internal courses of the meridians. Some acupuncturists even believe there are acupuncture points on the viscera which could be used effectively during surgical procedures. Perhaps more research will be done on this subject in the future.

Acupuncture should be thought of as a continually developing art with more points and techniques being discovered with experience, and scientific and technological progress. Acupuncture theory should be revised to conform with scientific evidence but should not be restricted by Western medical concepts.

REFERENCES FOR CHAPTER   4

1. Huard, P.; and Wong, M. *Chinese Medicine*. New York: McGraw–Hill Book Company, 1968.

2. Chou, T. S. (translator). *The Classical Chinese Medicine* (*Wan Han I Shieh*). Taipei, Taiwan: Kao–fung Publishing Company, 1960.

3. Chu, S. I.. "The Nature of Meridians and the Trend of Future Research." *The Journal of Chinese Medicine*. Peking, China, May 1958.

4. Ostrander, S.; and Schroeder, L. *Psychic Discoveries Behind the Iron Curtain*. Englewood Cliffs, New Jersey: Prentice–Hall, 1970.

5. Chu, L. *Contemporary Acupuncture and Moxibustion Therapy*. Hong Kong: Siaohwa Publishing Company, 1955.

6. Chou, A. C. "The Concept of Yin–Yang and Acupuncture Therapeutics." *Min Pao Monthly*. Hong Kong, October 1971.

7. Luh, S. Y.; and Chu, Y. K. *The Atlas and Explanations of the Commanding Loci of Chinese Acupuncture*. Taipei, Taiwan: Wen–Kuang Publishing Company, 1961.

chapter 5

NEUROPHYSIOLOGIC MECHANISMS IN ACUPUNCTURE

BIOCHEMICAL DISCOVERIES

Since 1975, there has been considerable evidence that acupuncture stimulates the nervous system to release enkephalins[1] and endorphins, naturally occurring analgesic substances.[2] This may explain why acupuncture can be an effective analgesic for surgery. It may also explain why and how acupuncture can relieve asthma, depression, and schizophrenia.

These morphine-like endogenous peptides have been found in the brain,[3] the cerebrospinal fluid,[4] the pituitary gland,[5] the adrenal glands, the gastro-intestinal tract and the blood.[6] There are many chemically different peptides with opiate-like activity found in different parts of the body. "Endorphin" is sometimes used as a general term to refer to all of them, including various enkephalins.[7] Their dis-

79

covery followed the observation that the body contained morphine-receptors, which could be rendered ineffective by the narcotic antagonists naloxone and naltrexone. Biochemists reasoned that if the body contained morphine–receptors, it must be capable of producing endogenous compounds with morphine–like activity.[8]

Unfortunately, few research biochemists know enough about acupuncture to perform it themselves or even evaluate the skill of acupuncturists they employ. And few skilled acupuncturists know much about biochemistry. In reading about attempts to compare acupuncture with transcutaneous electric stimulation (TES) in endorphin research, it is difficult to ascertain whether the TES was actually applied to acupuncture points or not.[9] There is great variation in TES equipment; some pierces the skin, and some does not. Nevertheless, it is significant that acupuncture without electric potentiation, electro-acupressure, and electro-acupuncture have all been demonstrated to increase endorphin levels in the spinal fluid, blood, and various other parts of the body.[10]

RELATIONSHIP OF THE NERVOUS SYSTEM TO THE VITAL ENERGY SYSTEM

Although the energy transmission system of the living body seems to be as independent as the digestive or circulatory systems, Chu[11], Kassil[12], and many others, have attempted to establish that the "material basis" of acupuncture therapy is primarily the nervous system. Since the nervous system controls all body functions, including the secretions of endocrine glands and brain cells, this seems to be a reasonable hypothesis. It should be understood, however, that acupuncture needles are not intended to pierce specific nervous tissues.

Bioelectric potential changes induced by acupuncture have been recorded from single cortical neurons.[13] This finding has led to the speculation that acupuncture–induced biopotential changes may diminish pain by inhibiting the nerve impulses produced by surgical incision.[14] The interaction between the inserted needle and the nerve fibers may be direct or indirect. Nerve fibers can be excited by mechanical stimulation or electrical stimulation with electro–acupuncture when an electric current is passed through the acupuncture needle. The acupuncture needle may influence the nervous system indirectly through the receptor cells which transform energy into nerve impulses propagating along the neural network.

OBJECTIVE EVIDENCE OF THE ENERGY
MERIDIAN SYSTEM

Acupuncture points have less electric resistance and higher electric potentials than surrounding areas of skin.[15] Instruments for precise location of acupuncture points are built on this principle. Surveys of acupuncture points with regard to their bioelectric properties have demonstrated that differences in the resistance and electric potential of acupuncture points can be precisely measured and sometimes used for diagnostic purposes.[16]

The connection between a visceral organ and its cutaneous projection may be explained in terms of embryology and neuroanatomy. The sensory inputs from cutaneous and visceral structures converge on the same neuron pool of the spinothalamic tract. The interaction between the visceral and the cutaneous structures may occur in the spinal cord and some other points along sensory pathways. This convergence–projection forms the neural basis of functional continuity between visceral and cutaneous structures that seems to be involved in acupuncture therapy.

REFERRED PAIN

Neural mechanisms are thought to be involved in referred visceral pain. Sensory inputs from the viscera may create an "irritable focus" in the spinal cord at the segment which they enter. The interaction between the visceral impulses and somatosensory impulses in the spinal cord results in the cutaneous projection of visceral reactions, according to C. L. Li.[17]

McLellan and Goodell[18] performed an experiment in which the ureter of a female patient was stimulated electrically near her kidney. Pain with typical references anteriorly along the border of the rectus muscle at the level of the umbilicus was reported. Stimulation of the kidney pelvis produced pain on her back at the junction of her ribs and vertebral column.

These findings suggest that these visceral structures and the areas where the pain was projected are connected by a converging nerve supply. The locations of referred pain produced by stimulating the ureteral–pelvic junction of the kidney as described by McLellan and Goodell coincide with part of the kidney meridian. The acupuncture points on this meridian, especially Kidney 11 to Kidney 21 on the abdominal wall, have been used for treating kidney and urinary tract diseases. The acupuncture point UB 23 (urinary bladder meridian) located on the back near the junction of the ribs and the vertebral column above the level of the umbilicus is designated as the kidney locus and is used for acupuncture therapy of kidney malfunctions. The kidney meridian (Ki) is continuous with the urinary bladder meridian (UB). Both meridians appear to be related to functions of the kidney, bladder, ureters, and other structures for water balance and the excretion of toxic elements in body fluid.

It is well known that coronary artery disease has a typical cutaneous pain projection, and referred pain in the arm and little finger has been useful in the diagnosis of coronary disease. Both the heart and vascular meridians pass along the arm. The acupuncture points along these two meridians can be used for relieving the pain of angina pectoris in cases where other therapy is inadequate or unavailable.

DISTRIBUTION OF ACUPUNCTURE POINTS

A general survey of the distribution of acupuncture points, especially those located on the trunk, shows segmental characteristics. The vertical meridians on the trunk are in general parallel to the midline sex and brain meridians. The head and face, however, are crowded with acupuncture points and meridians which change direction. The distribution of the acupuncture points on the extremities shows no segmental arrangements. This non–segmental distribution of some acupuncture points on the head, face, and extremities can probably be explained by the anatomic distribution of sensory root dermatomes.

A dermatome or sensory root field can be defined as the cutaneous area supplied with afferent fibers by a single posterior root of a specific nerve. These dermatomes were determined by hypesthesia resulting from ruptured intervertebral discs. In the original mapping by Keegan and Garnett [19] in the quadruped position (Figure 5–1), the dermatomes extend serially as bands from the cervical spine down the arm to the finger tips, from the thoracic spine to the chest and abdomen, and from the lumbar spine down the leg to the tips of the toes. The head and ear regions are supplied mainly by cranial nerves. Fibers from the first thoracic nerve pass down the arm to the tip of the fourth and fifth fingers. The visceral afferent and efferent nerves of the first thoracic segment supply the heart and lungs. A simple comparison between the distribution of dermatomes and the meridians indicates that the meridians also follow the serial distribution of dermatomes and may represent the overlapping areas with abundant nerve supplies.

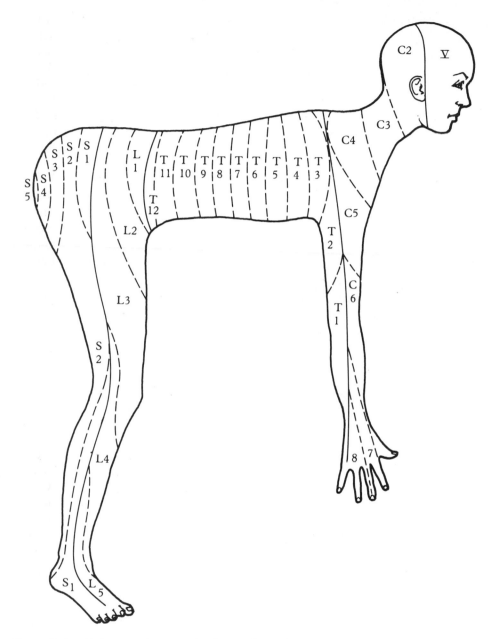

Figure 5–1.   Cutaneous innervation in quadruped position

The overlapping of dermatomes has been investigated by the method of "remaining sensibility." Sherrington[20] sectioned three roots above and three roots below the intact root to be studied, producing an island of sensitivity surrounded by an area of anesthesia. For example, at the level of the umbilicus, the horizontal line on the body wall represents the overlapping area of the ninth, tenth, and eleventh thoracic nerve roots. Along this horizontal line at the level of the umbilicus, one can locate acupuncture points Sx 8, Ki 16, St 24, Sp 15, GB 25, UB 46, UB 23, and Br 5. Thus, from the neuroanatomical and clinical studies of dermatomes, one may conclude that the acupuncture points and meridians represent the overlapping regions of adjacent nerve supplies or nerve plexuses.

NEUROPHYSIOLOGIC EXPLANATIONS

The functional continuity between cutaneous and visceral structures can be explained by our knowledge of neurophysiology. It is possible to consider the connections between the meridians as based on the complex neural circuits as a whole. The sequential flow of energy along the meridians postulated by the ancient Chinese, however, does not conform with our present understanding of nerve interaction and communication, although investigations of the therapeutic effects of acupuncture have shed some light on the nature of meridians.[21,22]

A consideration of some fundamental facts of neurophysiology is helpful in understanding the relationship between the nervous system and the energy meridian system. These two body systems are of course dependent on each other, and both systems are dependent on the circulatory, digestive, endocrine, and other body systems. The energy system works in cooperation with these as well as with the nervous system for homeostasis and good health.

Although the Korean scientist Kim Bong–Han[23] claims to have found special egg–shaped cells at acupuncture points and a microscopically demonstrable system of ducts containing nucleic acids in the meridian pathways, other researchers have been unable to find these and consider his reports erroneous. It seems more likely that the acupuncture points and meridian pathways are invisible and intangible like the electric waves of sound and light transmission for television. We should not confuse them with nerve fibers, sweat glands, lymphatic ducts, or other familiar structures.

BIOELECTRICITY

The single nerve cell has a bioelectric potential difference existing across its cell membrane, which is called the membrane potential, Em. The nerve membrane potential is caused by an unbalanced distribution of ions across the cell membrane. For example, mammalian nerve axons have the following ionic distributions:

	Intracellular		Extracellular
K^+	= 155 mM	K^+ =	4 mM
Na^+	= 12 mM	Na^+ =	145 mM
Cl^-	= 4 mM	Cl^- =	120 mM
mM	= millimoles/liter		

This unequal distribution is created by the selective membrane permeability and by an active transport process coupled to expenditure of metabolic energy. Although the sodium ion concentration is quite different on the two sides of the membrane, in the resting state (i.e., no action potential present) the membrane permeability to sodium is so low that the predominant membrane potential is due to the tendency of the potassium ion (K^+) to diffuse out of the cell. This results in a net negative charge inside the cell, and the membrane will therefore have an electric potential difference with the inside more negative than the outside. In most cells, the chloride ion diffuses passively in response to the membrane potential created by the potassium ion disequilibrium.[24]

The nerve membrane potential in the resting state can be calculated from the Nernst equation which relates the magnitude of the potential to the concentration of K^+ inside and outside the cell. This relationship is:

$$E_m = -\frac{RT}{zF} \ln \frac{K_i}{K_o} \qquad \text{Equation 1}$$

where K_i = concentration of K^+ inside the cell in mM/l (millimoles/liter)

K_o = concentration of K^+ outside the cell

E_m = membrane potential in millimoles per liter

R, T, z, F are constants that account for absolute temperature and charge of the ionic species, and allow expression of the electrochemical potential in the proper units.

ln = natural logarithm

At room temperature, the potential in millivolts, using logarithms to base 10, RT/zF = 61. Thus, for a cell with outside or extracellular concentration given in the table of K^+ of 4 mM/l, and inside concentration of approximately 155 mM/l, Equation 1 reduces to:

$$E_m = -61 \log \frac{155}{4} \qquad \textit{Equation 2}$$

$$E_m = -61 \log 39 = -61 \times 1.59 = -97 \text{ mv}$$

Lowering the extracellular concentration of K^+ will hyperpolarize the membrane or make the membrane potential more negative, while raising the extracellular concentration of K^+ will have the opposite effect; the membrane potential will become less negative. This is considered depolarization of the cell membrane. Thus, the effect of the ionic environment of the cell on membrane potential can be readily appreciated. Acupuncture might influence this.

Nerve fibers can be stimulated by mechanical, chemical, and electric factors. When the strength of stimulation exceeds the excitation threshold, membrane electric potential changes or nerve impulses are initiated. Nerve impulses can propagate along the nerve fiber and influence the activity or excitability of the nerve cell located in the spinal cord or the brain. Chemical and ionic changes, e.g., Na^+ influx and K^+ efflux, also accompany the electric phenomenon.[25] The possibility that acupuncture might influence some of these factors involved in bioelectric interchanges might be considered for future research.

SYNAPTIC TRANSMISSION

There is considerable evidence suggesting that almost all of the transmission of information between two neurons of higher vertebrates is electrochemical and therefore might be affected by acupuncture. Chemical transmission permits graded and finely controlled influence of different input information on the same neuron. In the central nervous system, some chemical transmitters are excitatory in nature, such as norepinephrine, dopamine and acetylcholine; some are inhibitatory in nature, such as serotonin.[26] The impulses of axonal terminals converging from different origins, may therefore release either excitatory or inhibitatory transmitters which have antagonistic effects on the same postsynaptic neuron. In summary, central synaptic transmission has the following characteristics:[27]

1. Convergence and divergence: A large number of presynaptic elements are involved. Presynaptic fibers carrying synaptic knobs to several cells is divergence. Many nerve terminals supplying the same cell is convergence.

2. Integration processes: The inhibitory and excitatory effects of presynaptic influences are usually local, graded, and subthreshold, making their integration possible.

3. Central inhibition and facilitation: The effects may be brought about by an influence on the presynaptic release of transmitters or by changing the responses to the transmitters.

Repetitive activity and stimulation may facilitate the function of any neural circuit through these mechanisms. Acupuncture may thus facilitate synaptic transmission.

MUSCLE RESPONSES

Muscles of the human body can be divided into three basic types: (1) skeletal muscle, (2) smooth muscle, and (3) cardiac muscle. The structures, functions, and electric properties of these muscle types are different from each other. The general characteristics of all muscle cells, however, are in some aspects similar to those of nerve cells because they all have electric membrane potentials caused by unequal ionic distributions across their membranes. The unequal ionic distributions are maintained by membrane selective permeability and the ionicly active transport system. The muscle cells, as well as the nerves, can be stimulated by electric, chemical, and mechanical factors, such as acupuncture.

Skeletal muscle fibers are capable of responding to an electric stimulus or nerve impulse in a few milliseconds. The functions of normal skeletal muscles are controlled by motor nerve terminals whose cell bodies are situated in the ventral horn of the spinal cord. Both cardiac muscle and smooth muscle are spontaneously active. The membrane electric activities control the rhythmic contractions of heart muscle, peristalsis, and sustained contractions of the uterus. Other factors, such as neurochemical agents, drugs, ionic exchanges, and the autonomic nerves, only modify the intrinsic activities of smooth muscle and cardiac muscle.[28] For example, stimulation of the vagus nerve can reduce the heart rate. The effect of the autonomic nervous system is to modify spontaneous activity. Acupuncture may affect autonomic nerve transmission.

Vagal inhibition is brought about by a membrane hyperpolarization (increased electric potential) due to increased potassium ion permeability produced by acetylcholine released from the vagus nerve endings. Stimulation of the sympathetic nerve supply can accelerate the heart rate by increasing the rate of its pacemaker depolarization. An intact heart *in situ*, isolated from all nerve supply and chemical influences in the blood, can continue to beat at a normal rate for hours, however.

Smooth muscle electric activities and muscle contractions are also regulated and influenced by the autonomic nervous system and the ionic medium of the internal environment. For example, increased calcium concentration (two times normal plasma concentration) changes the electric activity of mammalian intestinal muscle from slow wave activity with one cycle lasting five to ten seconds into trains of action potentials with one cycle lasting five to 100 milliseconds.[29] Changes in electric properties of smooth muscles also modify the tonus and function of the digestive tract. When the muscle membrane is depolarized (membrane electric potential reduced in amplitude), calcium ions are released from the sarcoplasmic reticulum and Z lines to initiate muscle contraction. Acupuncture may thereby influence activity of the digestive system by causing changes in the electric potentials of muscle membranes.

The fine structures of contractile filaments in smooth muscle cells and cardiac muscle cells have not been clearly demonstrated. It is possible, however, that calcium ions released by membrane depolarization control muscle contraction and tonus in all types of muscles. Membrane potentials of nerve cells and muscles are all determined by the distribution of ions in body fluids and tissues. Blood plasma concentrations of Ca^+, Na^+, and K^+ have an important influence on the nervous system and muscles. If acupuncture affects these ion concentrations, it can have a significant influence on muscle function.

The electric membrane potentials of the muscle cells at rest determine the excitability of the muscles. Muscle cells with an abnormally high amplitude of membrane potentials (hyperpolarization) or an excessive negative charge inside the membrane tend to have lower excitability. Muscle cells with slightly low membrane potentials (hypopolarization) tend to be more excitable. The electric properties of smooth muscle cells influence biochemical and digestive functions. Extreme hyperpolarization tends to inhibit the normal mobility and function of visceral muscle cells. A balance of charge distributions inside and outside of the muscle cells is essential to maintain the normal activities of the visceral organs. Because of its ability to produce changes in membrane electric potentials, acupuncture may be able to restore this balance if it has been upset by internal or external environmental factors.

In the heart, the sinusoid nodal area, or the pacemaker region, has lower membrane potentials; the cells are spontaneously active, and the electric activities of the pacemaker cells control the rhythm of heart beats.

Skeletal muscle cells have high amplitudes of resting membrane potentials (90–100 millivolts). This type of muscle cell is not spontaneously active. The skeletal muscle cells are activated by the chemical transmitters released from the nerve terminals to excite the muscle membrane by depolarization.[30]

It is evident that electric potentials have an important influence on the activity and function of all types of muscle cells. Even the kidney tubule system has electric potentials across the tubular walls. All human cells, in fact, have resting membrane potentials, and their activities are regulated by electric potential changes. Hyperpolarization (an excess of negative charges inside the cell) tends to inhibit normal activities. Slight hypopolarization (slight reduction of membrane potentials) tends to enhance activities. The excitability of a muscle or nerve cell is related to its action potential or a shift of the membrane electric potential from negative to positive.[31] The effect of acupuncture on various types of body cells, however, has not yet been clearly evaluated.

ELECTRO-ACUPUNCTURE FINDINGS

According to some clinical observations and research reports on electro–acupuncture, the acupuncture points on the meridian leading to a hyperactive organ all bear positive electric charges.[32] This condition is considered *Yang*. When the organ is hypoactive, an excess of negative charges in its meridian and acupuncture points can be detected. This condition is considered *Yin*. Electro–acupuncture techniques use weak current to neutralize the excess negative charges of hypoactive meridians (stimulation or tonification) or to supply negative charges to hyperactive meridians and visceral organs (sedation).

This simplistic concept of organ malfunction, however, has not been accepted by American physicians. We know that visceral organs and peripheral parts of the body can malfunction and produce distressing symptoms without being either underactive or overactive. It seems more likely that acupuncture, with or without electric potentiation, mediates its effects on specific organs through the autonomic nervous system and parts of the brain and other tissues which produce endorphins.[33] Increasing endogenous opiate–like compounds explains how acupuncture relieves pain, depression, and allergies. This does not, however, explain how acupuncture can relieve paresis or neurogenic sensory organ malfunction.

The bioelectric properties of all tissue cells and the functions of membrane potentials in different types of cells indicate the vital role of bioelectric energy communication and control among different organs and systems for the preservation of life processes. Classical acupuncture theory is based on the concepts of *Yin* (negativity) and *Yang* (positivity), the circulation of blood and *Chi* (vital energy). To find a scientific explanation for these concepts, we should attempt to gain a better understanding of the distribution and circulation of bioelectric energy in the human body.

KIRLIAN PHOTOGRAPHY

Experiments using high frequency photographic techniques to study energy distributions in the human body carried out in Russia by the Kirlians and similar studies performed by Tiller[34] and others in the United States have demonstrated the distribution of bioluminescence along the meridian lines and discharges from the meridian *loci* or acupuncture points. The nature of the bioluminescence and energy photographed in high frequency electric fields is not clearly understood. The possibility that there are special acupuncture receptor cells which transform biochemical energy into nerve impulses (electric energy) might be considered but does not seem likely in spite of Kim's[23] claim that he discovered such cells.

GATE CONTROL THEORY

Recent reports from acupuncture research institutes and neurophysiologic laboratories suggest that acupuncture therapy involves the somatosensory nerves and the autonomic nervous system. A needle inserted in a chosen acupuncture point can eliminate pain in a particular area just as local infiltration of procaine, or other local anesthetic agent, blocks impulse conduction of somatosensory nerves. This finding suggests that the afferent nerve fibers of somatic sensations are directly involved in the chain of events by which acupuncture produces pain relief.

Receptors of the somatosensory nerves are located in the skin. These receptors have been classified as follows: (1) Pacini's corpuscle for gross tactile sensation, (2) Meissner's corpuscle for fine tactile sensation, (3) Ruffini's end–organ for heat perception, (4) Krause's end–bulb for cold perception, and (5) the free nerve endings for pain perception.

One explanation for the mechanisms of the analgesic effect of acupuncture suggests that acupuncture–induced impulses transmitted in nerve fibers normally responsible for tactile sensations can inhibit the pain sensations transmitted by pain fibers. These small myelinated fibers are free nerve terminals which transmit pain sensations to the brain. C. L. Li [17] of the National Institutes of Health has completed a study on the interaction between the bioelectric potentials conducted in the small pain fibers (diameters smaller than 2–3 microns) and the electric responses of large myelinated fibers (diameters larger than 3 microns), which are related to muscle function, autonomic function, proprioceptive, tactile, and temperature sensations. His evidence also suggests that bioelectric responses carried in the tactile or proprioceptive fibers can inhibit the pain response. Li's study indicates that the bioelectric potentials carried in pain fibers and tactile fibers have some inhibitory interaction even at the peripheral level.

Acupuncture may stimulate nerve fibers or somatosensory receptors in the vicinity. The receptors for tactile sensations, namely, Pacini's corpuscles and Meissner's corpuscles, may be involved. Ruffini's end–organ for heat perception is receptive to the heat which is often applied to potentiate acupuncture therapy. Pain fibers enter the spinal cord through the dorsal root ganglia. These fibers pass Lissauer's zone and synapse with cells in the dorsal horn; the axons of these cells become the lateral spinothalamic tract and terminate in a specific sensory relay nucleus, the nucleus ventralis posterior lateralis of the thalamus, and then project to the sensory cortex of the brain. Fibers from Pacini's corpuscles terminate in the dorsal column of the spinal cord, and fibers from Meissner's corpuscles proceed along different pathways after entering the dorsal root ganglia. Both ascend to higher nervous centers. [35]

Primary afferent collaterals in the spinal cord are distributed to the dorsal horn and substantia gelatinosa, which has been considered a gate control for pain sensation. [36]

Other collaterals are reflex motor nerves extending to the ventral horn, where the nerve cells for motor functions are located. Fibers from pain receptors enter the dorsal root ganglia along with fibers from Meissner's corpuscles and ascend in nearby columns to converge in the ventral posterior nucleus of the thalamus. It is possible, therefore, for somatosensory sensations to interact at different levels of the nervous system, from the peripheral to higher centers.

Somatosensory receptors function as transducers to transform mechanical, chemical, and thermal stimulations to electric energy. Generator potentials or bioelectric potential changes have been recorded from some receptors.

The gate theory of explaining how acupuncture produces analgesia for surgery may have some validity, but seems less plausible than theories regarding the release of endorphins from acupuncture stimulation. None of these theories, however, accounts for the lasting relief of chronic pain or the restoration of function achieved by a series of acupuncture treatments.

MECHANISM OF ENERGIZATION (Te-Chi)

Some neurophysiologists reject the idea that somatosensory receptors and nerves are involved in acupuncture, but the energization (*Te–Chi*) sensations patients experience during acupuncture treatment suggest that the somatosensory system may play a part in initiating the complicated events of the physiologic and biochemical regulations apparently produced by acupuncture. According to classical Chinese medical books and modern investigations, the sensation of energization (*Te–Chi*) is the key to the success of acupuncture therapy. When a needle is inserted exactly into an acupuncture point, a person feels a sensation of heaviness, fullness, and tingling there. He should also feel as if a mild electric current is passing along the meridian on which the point is located toward the organ after which it is named. It is, therefore, unlikely that a patient would confuse skilled acupuncture with needles at random for double-blind experiments.

Electronic point–finding instruments can be used to distinguish between acupuncture points and surrounding areas of skin. Most of these instruments produce a special sound and the *Te–Chi* sensation when their probes are directly over an acupuncture point.

Although the sensations of *Te-Chi* follow the course of the meridians, there is considerable similarity between the courses of most of the meridians and nerve pathways. Some observers believe that the somatosensory system and its interactions with the visceral or autonomic nervous system may play an important role in the mechanism of *Te–Chi* or energization sensation.

AUTONOMIC INFLUENCES

In search of a possible mechanism of acupuncture, many investigators, including Gerald L. Looney,[37] have come to the conclusion that acupuncture exerts its therapeutic effects on the body by influencing the autonomic nervous system.

The autonomic nervous system innervates smooth muscle, cardiac muscle, and glands. By influencing the muscular and glandular components of the visceral organs, blood vessels, and other structures, the autonomic nervous system regulates the functions of vital systems to cope with emergency situations and to restore and maintain an optimal internal environment for life processes.

Autonomic nervous control can modify the activity of the structure innervated without changing the intrinsic and spontaneous nature of the visceral organ. Sections of human intestines can be kept active for hours in a 37°C incubator with oxygen supply in a saline medium. The basic feature of autonomic regulation is a modification of the bioelectric potentials of the innervated muscle or glandular cells. The chemical transmitters acetylcholine and norepinephrine are mediators which have antagonistic actions to exert a finely graded control of the electric responses.[38] Using the pacemaker cells of the heart as an example, one may present a scheme to explain the antagonistic influences of the sympathetic and parasympathetic innervations.

Autonomic Regulation of the Heart

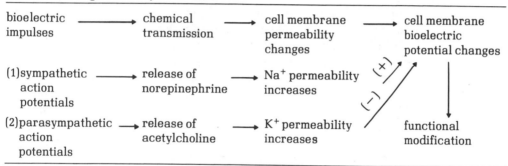

The influence of the vagus nerve (parasympathetic) is to increase the membrane potential amplitude and to reduce the heart rate, while membrane depolarization tends to increase the heart rate. Electric potential changes of heart muscle cells control the rate and strength of heart beats. Considering the extensive influence of the autonomic nervous system on the vital organs and glandular secretions, there is good reason to think that acupuncture acts on the autonomic nervous system, perhaps by influencing the levels of neurochemicals.

EFFECTS ON THE BRAIN

Numerous investigations and reports have provided evidence that various subcortical structures lying at the base of the brain play an important part in emotion, consciousness, memory, motivation, and control of body physiology and chemistry. Moruzzi and Magoun [39] demonstrated in 1949 that the activity of the reticular formation of the brain (RF) is essential for consciousness. Other investigators have shown that auditory and somatic sensory inputs exert their influence on the cortex by way of the ascending reticular system, which receives collaterals throughout the midbrain and projects impulses to the cortex from the nonspecific reticular nuclei of the thalamus.[40]

The nucleus reticularis has been considered as the final relay nucleus of the thalamus, and the projection to the cortex has been termed the "non–specific projection system."

After discovery of the important functions of the reticular formation, a series of findings clarified the intrinsic roles of the limbic system. Kluver and Bucy[41] found that drastic disturbances in emotion, memory, and behavior were produced by bilateral removal of temporal lobes in monkeys. Penfield[42] demonstrated the functions of the temporal lobes by direct electric stimulation in conscious human beings during brain surgery. Papez[43] mapped the complex neural circuit provided by the hippocampus, fornix, mammillary bodies, mammillothalamic tracts, anterior nucleus of the thalamus, and cingulate gyrus. He suggested that this circuit is primarily concerned with the control of emotion and not merely olfaction.

Within the limbic system, the amygdala and the hippocampus control the connections between the temporal neocortex and subcortical limbic systems. The amygdala, like the hippocampus, is sensitive to a wide variety of afferent inflow. The most effective stimuli are touch and sciatic nerve stimulation.[44] In view of the key importance of these two structures in controlling autonomic regulation and mental functions, one is reminded again of the possible antagonistic interaction between touch sensation and the conscious feeling of pain.

Within the complex neural circuits of the limbic system, one important circuit for autonomic regulation via the hypothalamus may be diagrammed as follows:

(HC) Hippocampus ⟶ Septal region ⟶ Hypothalamus ⟶ Reticular formation ⟶ HC

Amygdala ⟶ Septal region ⟶ Hypothalamus ⟶ Reticular formation ⟶ Amygdala

Autonomic regulation

Endorphins with morphine-like activity were isolated from the hypothalamus in 1975.[45] Nerve terminals containing dopamine, norepinephrine, and serotonin, as well as acetylcholine, have also been found in the hypothalamus.[46] The complexity of chemical transmitters involved may represent the different sources of control and influence on the neurons in this region. Excitatory and inhibitory chemical transmitters released from different nerve terminals converging on the same neuron may exert a graded and antagonistic influence on the bioelectric outputs of the hypothalamus to the lower autonomic nervous pathways.

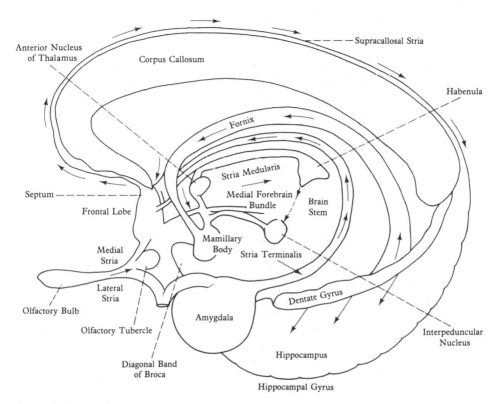

Figure 5-2.   Limbic brain connections

Neurons in the amygdala and the hippocampus receive both inhibitory nerve terminals using serotonin as the chemical transmitter and excitatory inputs using catecholamines as the transmitters. The excitatory terminals can be traced back to their cell bodies in the midbrain reticular formation, and their axons travel primarily in the medial forebrain bundles. Swedish neurophysiologists Anden, Dahlstrom, and their associates came to these conclusions in 1966.[47]

The importance of the amygdala and the hippocampus in controlling body physiology and chemistry is stressed by the endocrine studies of Kawakami et al.[48] Stimulation of both structures increases corticosteroid secretion. Exogenous corticosteroid, however, suppresses the activity of the amygdala and enhances the influence of the hippocampus. ACTH has the opposite effect. The amygdala and hippocampus are also involved in the control of ovarian function. Stimulation of the centromedian amygdala gives rise to ovulation, and stimulation of the dorsal hippocampus increases progesterone production by the ovary. All these changes are accompanied by changes in the bioelectric activities of the two centers. (See Figure 5-3.)

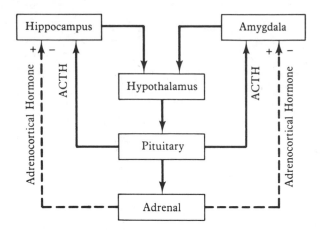

Figure 5–3.   Feedback control of adrenal cortical secretions

Based on the above considerations, acupuncture stimulation of nerve fibers conducting touch and proprioceptive sensations may alter the activities of the amygdala and hippocampus to enhance normal defense mechanisms against disease and emotional trauma. This may be one important link in the overall mechanism of acupuncture.

Acetylcholinesterase is found in the amygdala, hippocampus, and associated fiber tracts in the limbic systems, as well as in the caudate and putamen. The functions of the cholinergic system of the brain are not well understood, but these recent findings point out the importance of the basal ganglia of the brain and the seriousness of damaging them by long-term ingestion of phenothiazines and other tranquilizing drugs.

The somatosensory projections of the subcortical ganglia and their interactions with the visceral and interoceptive inputs may play an important part in the general effects of acupuncture. The reduction of dyskinesia and Parkinsonian symptoms by acupuncture treatments supports this possibility.

BIOCHEMICAL EFFECTS OF ACUPUNCTURE

Evidence that acupuncture can increase the endorphins in blood, spinal fluid, and various tissues has made the analgesic, antidepressant, and antiallergic effects of acupuncture more understandable.[49]

Other biochemical effects of acupuncture have been reported by Cracium, Toma, and Turdeanu.[50] They measured phagocytic and fibrinolytic activities in human subjects before and after acupuncture. They found that acupuncture increased phagocytic activity by 55.6%

and fibrinolytic activity by 79%. To explain these results, they reasoned that acupuncture caused stimulation of the hypothalamic and diencephalic centers which regulate phagocytic and fibrinolytic activities in the blood via the hypothalamo-medullar pathway and the sympathetic adrenergic system.

Tykochinskaia[51] studied the effects of acupuncture on leucocytes by inserting a needle at acupuncture point Stomach 36 (Tsusanli) for 30 minutes. In most cases, this induced a biphasic reaction in the form of leucopenia for 15 to 30 minutes following acupuncture and a subsequent leucocytosis which reached its highest level after three hours. After 24 hours, leucocyte counts returned to normal.

At the Sansi Acupuncture Symposium in 1959, C. K. Yang[52] reported that, during acupuncture treatment at St 36, leucocyte counts increased more than 50% and reached a peak of 70% increase 2 to 3 hours after acupuncture. In 24 hours, the number of leucocytes partially recovered to 30% above the control values prior to the acupuncture. Needles inserted at non-acupuncture points did not have the same effects. Blockade of the sciatic nerves by local anesthesia or general anesthesia abolished the effects of acupuncture at St 36 on the changes in leucocyte counts, according to Yang.

C. Y. Kao[53] demonstrated that acupuncture at St 36 and Colon 11 transiently decreased the content of SH (sulfhydryl) groups in the blood with recovery completed in 8 hours. The content of SH groups in the cerebral cortex, liver, kidney, and skeletal muscle tissues increased markedly after acupuncture. For example, the activity of the enzyme succinodehydrogenase increased after five or more acupuncture treatments applied to points Brain 16 (Fenfu), Urinary Bladder 19 (Tanshu) and 23 (Shenshu), and Stomach 36 (Tsusanli).

The influence of acupuncture on endocrine secretion and immunologic reactions has been studied in China, Japan, and the United States. J. Y. Li[54] stimulated the pituitary-adrenal system in rabbits with acupuncture. The weight of the adrenal gland increased, and the adrenal cortex increased in thickness. Yang-Ming Chu and Lewis F. Affronti of George Washington University did research on the effects of acupuncture on immune responses in sensitized guinea pigs.[55]

All secretions of the adrenal glands are controlled by the activity of amygdaloid nuclei, the pituitary gland, the endogenous concentrations of ACTH, and adrenocorticosteroid, according to the feedback mechanism proposed by Kawakami et. al.[56] Symthies and Adey[57] also described the key importance of the amygdaloid nucleus in regulating adrenal gland secretion. Stimulating the sciatic nerve increased amygdaloid nucleus activity as measured by bioelectric potential changes in their experiments.

EFFECTS OF ACUPUNCTURE ON PAIN SYNDROMES AND THE NERVOUS SYSTEM

Especially since 1960, recognition of the therapeutic values of acupuncture for pain syndromes has been established by clinical observations in many countries. Valery[58] in France in 1966, Vacek[59] in Czechoslovakia in 1969, and Kormeichuk and Zingerman[60] in Russia in 1968 reported the analgesic effects of acupuncture on facial neuralgia. Hyodo[61] in Japan in 1968 wrote about the treatment of whiplash injury by electro-acupuncture. Acupuncture was reported as effective for treating severe and recurrent radiculitis by Demidenko[62] in Russia in 1961. Plethysmographic vasomotor responses in lumbosacral root syndromes were registered both after specific stimulation by acupuncture and after non-specific stimuli by Czechoslovakian scientists[63] in 32 cases in 1964. They found that vasomotor responses were restored to normal after acupuncture.

Treatment of post-tonsillectomy pain by acupuncture was compared with chemical analgesia by Odehnal[64] in Czechoslovakia in 1970. He concluded that acupuncture treatments were safe and could be used in cases where the administration of drugs was not recommended.

In 1968, parallel investigations were conducted in China on 88 people to study the effects of acupuncture on the functions of the central nervous system.[65] The results showed that strong stimulation inhibited the electric activities of the cerebral cortex (as revealed by electroencephalograms) in subjects with neurologic disorders. The same strong stimulus also had an inhibitory effect on healthy individuals, but the effect was less and of shorter duration. These findings suggest that the effects of acupuncture on the central nervous system depend on the strength of stimulation as well as on the physiological condition of individuals.

REGULATORY EFFECTS OF ACUPUNCTURE

The overall influence of acupuncture apparently is regulatory, and is most effective in pathological cases. The effects of acupuncture as shown on electroencephalograms have been studied by Chang[66] and Kassil.[12] Both reported that the amplitude of patients' frontal-occipital EEG alpha waves was increased. An increase in the synchronization of the alpha rhythm and the appearance of theta rhythm were noticed while the acupuncture needles were inserted. Kassil suggested that the general reaction of acupuncture was brought about by nonspecific action on the higher regions of the central nervous system through the reticular system of the brainstem.

The regulatory action of acupuncture on the autonomic nervous system was studied by R.S. Wei[67] in 1952. He found that acupuncture could increase the excitability of the sympathetic nervous system and sedate the parasympathetic nervous system. He studied the therapeutic effect of acupuncture on nerve regeneration by experimental sectioning of the sixth lumbar roots of rabbits. The contractile functions of denervated muscles recovered gradually after acupuncture treatments. Denervated muscles of rabbits which did not receive acupuncture treatment remained nonfunctional. Wei suggested that acupuncture might stimulate the regeneration of sectioned nerve fibres.

L. Y. Tang[68] used X-ray multiple-exposure techniques to study gastric peristalsis before and after acupuncture in 50 patients. Acupuncture applied at point St 36 on the leg was found to be the most effective for reducing the magnitude of stomach peristalsis.

Other Chinese scientists found that acupuncture applied at points Sex 14, 17, and 22, or Colon 4 increased the magnitude of gastric and esophageal peristalsis. J. B. Yu[69] reported in 1959 that during coma, when stomach peristalsis completely disappeared, acupuncture applied to points Stomach 36 and Urinary Bladder 21 (*Weishu* or stomach locus) were most effective in restoring normal stomach peristalsis and secretions.

Much more research needs to be done to determine exactly what role the nervous system plays in the regulatory and analgesic effects of acupuncture on various body tissues.

REFERENCES FOR CHAPTER   5

1. Mendelson, G. "The Role of Enkephalin in the Mechanism of Acupuncture Analgesia in Man." *Medical Hypotheses* 2(4)(July-Aug. 1977): 144–145.

2. Sjölund, Bengt; and Eriksson, Margareta. "Electro-Acupuncture and Endogenous Morphines." *Lancet* 2 (Nov. 1976): 1085.

3. Snyder, Solomon H. "The Opiate Receptor and Morphine-like Peptides in the Brain." *American Journal of Psychiatry* 135(6)(June 1978): 645–652.

4. Sjölund, Bengt.; Terenius, L.; and Eriksson, M. "Increased Cerebrospinal Fluid Levels of Endorphins after Electro-Acupuncture." *Acta Physiologica Scandinavica.* 100(3)(July 1977): 382–384.

5. Goldstein, A. "Opiod Peptides (Endorphins) in Pituitary and Brain." *Science* 193 (1976): 1081–1086.

6. Pert, C. B.; Pert, A.; and Tallman, J. F. "Isolation of a Novel Endogenous Opiate Analgesic from Human Blood.", Proceedings of the National Academy of Science, U.S.A. 73 (1976): 2226–2230.

7. Miller, Richard J. "The Potential of Endorphins." *Behavioral Medicine* (May 1979) 30–33.

8. Hughes, John. "Isolation of an Endogenous Compound from the Brain with Pharmacological Properties Similar to Morphine." *Brain Research* 88: (Amsterdam 1975): 295–308.

9. Fox, J. Elisabeth; and Melzak, Ronald. "Transcutaneous Electrical Stimulation and Acupuncture: Comparison of Treatment for Low-Back Pain." *Pain* 2 (Amsterdam 1976): 141–148.

10. Pomeranz, B.; Cheng, R.; and Law, P. "Acupuncture Reduces Electrophysiological and Behavioral Responses to Noxious Stimuli: Pituitary is Implicated." *Experimental Neurology* 54 (1977): 172–178.

11. Chu, Lien. *Contemporary Acupuncture and Moxibustion Therapy*, Ch. II, *The Mechanism of Acupuncture Therapy*, pp. 11–15, Siaohwa Pub. Co., Hong Kong, 1955.

12. Kassil, G. M. "Mechanism of Therapeutic Effect of Acupuncture." *Vestnik Akademic Meditsmkikh.* NAUK, Moscow 16(3) (1961): 37–47.

13. Hyodo, M. "Relationship between Nerve Blocking for Pain Relief at Acupuncture Points in Oriental Medicine." *Japanese Journal of Anasthesiology* 16 (1967): 523–534.

14. Chu, S. I. "The Nature of Meridians and the Trend of Future Research." *The Journal of Chinese Medicine* May 1958.

15. Su, L. S. "Research on Meridians." *The Journal of Chinese Medicine* Oct. 1958.

16. Manaka, Y. "On Certain Electrical Phenomena for the Interpretation of Chi in Chinese Acupuncture." *American Journal of Chinese Medicine.* 3(1) Jan. 1975.

17. Li, C. L. "Neurological Basis of Pain and Its Possible Relationship to Acupuncture-Analgesia." *Journal of Chinese Medicine* 1 (1973) 61.

18. McLellan, A. M.; and Goodell, H. *Research Publication of the Association of Neurological and Mental Diseases* 23 (1943): 252–262.

19. Keegan, J. D.; and Garnett, F. D. *Anatomical Records*, 102 (1948): 409–437.

20. Sherrington, C. S. *Philadelphia Transactions*, B 190 (1898): 450186.

21. Luh, S. Y. "Research on the Relationship between the Theory of Meridians and Acupuncture Therapeutics." *The Journal of Chinese Medicine.*, July and October 1948.

22. Sun, J. C. "The Theory of Meridians and Acupuncture Therapeutics." *Modern Chinese Medicine and Therapeutics.* Peking, December 1957.

23. Kim, Bong-Han. *Proceedings Academy of Kyungrak*, #2, Pyongyank, Korea: Medical Science Press, 1965.

24. Woodbury, F. W. "The Cell Membrane: Ionic and Potential Gradients and Active Transport." in *Physiology and Biophysics.* Edited by T. C. Ruch and H. D. Patton. Philadelphia: W. B. Saunders Co., 1966.

25. Hodgkin, A. L. "The Ionic Basis of Electrical Activity in Nerve and Muscle." *Biological Review* 26 (1951): 339–409.

26. McLellan, H. *Synaptic Transmission.* Philadelphia: W. B. Saunders Co., 1963.

27. Snyder, S. H., et al., "Uptake and Subcellular Localization of Neurotransmitters in the Brain." *International Review of Neurobiology* 3 (1970): 127–159.

28. Katz, B. *Nerve, Muscle and Synapse.* New York: McGraw-Hill, 1966.

29. Liu, J. H.; Prosser, C. L.; and Job, D. "Ionic Dependence of Intestinal Smooth Muscle." *Journal of American Physiology* 1969.

30. Nastuk, W. L. "Neuromuscular Transmission." *The American Journal of Medicine* 19(5) (1955): 633–638.

31. Guyton, Arthur C. *Textbook of Medical Physiology.* 5th ed. Philadelphia: W. B. Saunders Co., 1976.

32. Shiao, U. S. "The Conditions of the Meridians Studied by Skin Electrical Resistance." *The Journal of Chinese Medicine* February 1958.

33. Liao, Sung J. "Recent Advances in the Understanding of Acu-

puncture." *Yale Journal of Biology and Medicine* 51(1) (January–February 1978): 55–65.

34. Tiller, William A. *Some Energy Field Observations of Man and Nature.* Stanford, California: Stanford University, 1972.

35. Ruch, T. C. "Pathophysiology of Pain." Chapter 16 in *Physiology and Biophysics.* Edited by T. C. Ruch and P. D. Patton. New York: W. B. Saunders Co., 1966.

36. Melzack, R.; and Wall, P. D. "Pain Mechanisms: A New Theory." *Science* 150 (1965): 971–9.

37. Looney, Gerald L. "Autonomic Theory of Acupuncture." *American Journal of Chinese Medicine* 2(2) (1974): 332–333.

38. MacLean, P. D. "Implications of Microelectrode Findings on Exteroceptive Inputs to the Limbic Cortex." In *Limbic System Mechanisms and Autonomic Function,* edited by Charles H. Hockman. Springfield, Missouri: Thomas Pub. Co., 1972.

39. Moruzzi, G.; and Magoun, H. W. "Electroencephalography." *Clinical Neuro-physiology* 1 (1949): 455–473.

40. Gastaut, H. "Some Aspects of the Neurophysiological Basis of Conditioned Reflexes and Behavior." In *The Neurophysiological Basis of Behavior,* edited by G. E. W. Wolstenholme and C. M. O'Connor, pp. 255–72. London: Ciba, 1958.

41. Kluver, H; and Bucy, P. C. *American Journal of Physiology* 119 (1937): 352.

42. Penfield, W.; and Pratt, P. *Brain* 86 (1963): 696.

43. Papez, J. W. *Archives of Neurology and Psychiatry* 38 (1937): 725.

44. Smythies, J. R. *Brain Mechanisms and Behavior.* 2nd ed.. New York: Academic Press, 1970.

45. Pasternak, G. W.; Goodman, R.; and Snyder, S. N. "An Endogenous Morphine-Like Factor in Mammalian Brain." *Life Science* 16 (1975): 1765–1769.

46. Moore, R. Y. "Brain Lesions and Amine Metabolism." *International Review of Neurobiology* 13 (1970): 67091.

47. Anden, N. E.; Dahlstrom, A.; et al., "Ascending Monamine Neurons to the Telencephalon and Diencephalon." *Acta Physiologica Scandinavica* 67 (1966): 313–326.

48. Kawakami, M.; Seto, K.; et al. *Progress in Brain Research* 27 (1967): 69.

49. Wei, Ling Y. "Scientific Advances in Acupuncture." *American Journal of Chinese Medicine* 7(1) (Spring 1978): 53–75.

50. Cracium, T.; Toma, C.; and Turdeanu, V. "Neurohumoral Modification after Acupuncture." *American Journal of Acupuncture* 21 (1973): 67–70.

51. Tykochinskaia, E. O. "Acupuncture as a Method of Reflex Therapy." *Voprosy Psikhiatrii i Nerropathologii* 7 (1960): 249–260.

52. Yang, C. K. "Clinical Report." *Sansi Acupuncture Symposium.* 1959.

53. Kao, C. Y. "Effects of Acupuncture on the Activity of Succino-Dehydrogenase." *Shenyang Medical Journal* 1, 1958.

54. Li, J. Y. "The Effects of Acupuncture on the Activity of the Rabbit Adrenal Gland." *Shenyang Medical Journal* 1, 1958.

55. Chu, Yang-Ming; and Affronti, Lewis F. "Preliminary Observations on the Effects of Acupuncture on Immune Responses in Sensitized Rabbits and Guinea Pigs." *American Journal of Chinese Medicine* 3(2) (1975): 151–163.

56. Kawakami, M.; Seto, K.; et al. "Feedback Control of the Adrenal Cortical Secretion." *Progressive Brain Research* 27 (1967): 69.

57. Smythies, J. R.; and Adey, W. R. *Brain Mechanisms and Behavior*, Chapter II, pp. 31–33, 1959.

58. Valery, L. P. "Homeopathy and Acupuncture: Facial Neuralgia." *Chirurgien-Dentiste de France* (Paris) 36 (July 1966): 41–43.

59. Vacek, J.; Tuhacek, J.; et al: "The Correlation of Palm-mental Reflex and Distant Points of Acupuncture." *Askoslovenska Neurologie* (Prague) 32 (May 1969): 146–150.

60. Kormeichuk, A. G.; and Zingerman, V. "Experience in Acupuncture Treatment of Patients with Involvement of the Facial Nerve." *Vrachnebnoe Delo* 11 (November 1968): 84–87.

61. Hyodo, M. "The New Therapy of Whiplash Injury by Electric Acupuncture." *Japanese Journal of Anesthesiology* 17 (June 1968) 573–579.

62. Demidenko, T. D. "Effect of Acupuncture on the Course of Severe and Recurrent Radiculitis." *Voprosy Psikhiatrii I Nervopatologii* 7 (1961): 261–267.

63. Figar, S., et al. "Vasomotor Responses to Acupuncture in Lumbosacral Root Syndrome." *Ceskoslovenska Neurologie* 27 (July 1964): 251–255.

64. Odehnal, F. "A Comparative Study of the Analgesic Effect of Acupuncture with the Analgesic Effect of Some Chemical Analgesics in Patients after Tonsillectomy." *Ceskoslovenska Otolaryngologie* 19 (August 1970): 161–165.

65. Tong, C. T., et al., "The Influences of Acupuncture Therapeutics on the Central Nervous System." *Journal of Chinese Medicine* 5, 1968.

66. Chang, C. L. "Clinical Observations and Investigations on the Effects of Acupuncture and Moxibustion Therapeutics." *Journal of Chinese Medicine* 6, 1956.

67. Wei, R. S. "Investigations on the Mechanisms and Therapeutic Effects of Acupuncture Treatments." *China North East Medical Journal* 2, 1952.

68. Tang, L. Y. "The Influence of Acupuncture on Stomach Peristalsis." *Journal of Chinese Radiation Research* 8 (April 1960): 90–94.

69. Yu, J. B. "X-ray Observations of the Effects of Acupuncture Applied to Functions of the Stomach." *Jiangsi Chinese Medicine and Pharmacy*, April, 1959.

chapter 6

TEACHING ACUPUNCTURE TO AMERICANS

Americans with good backgrounds in basic medical sciences should be able to master the art of acupuncture without learning much about Chinese philosophy. Although it is interesting to be aware of the ancient Chinese concepts and laws on which acupuncture is based, it is not advisable to ignore previous medical training while studying or performing acupuncture. The student of acupuncture should try to integrate the scientific knowledge he already has with what he learns about acupuncture.

Some English and American physicians have written books and given lectures on acupuncture which make little or no attempt to reconcile it with modern science. When questioned about this, they say that Oriental and Western thinking are irreconcilable, that while practicing or discussing acupuncture, they put aside their Western medical training and try to operate within the framework of ancient

Chinese medical concepts. This is a mistake. Scientific truth is the same the world over. Both acupuncture theory and modern Western medical theory can benefit from being corrected in accordance with scientific discoveries.

ENERGY MERIDIAN SYSTEM

Chinese acupuncture theory does not seem to conform to current American scientific standards. As the concept of biopotential is used by Americans for such diagnostic procedures as electrocardiograms, electroencephalograms, and biofeedback, however, it becomes increasingly difficult to deny the Chinese concept of a body energy system on which acupuncture is based. Although Americans know that these standard American diagnostic procedures utilizing body energy do not involve attempts at piercing nerves, they seem to have great difficulty accepting the idea that acupuncture does not aim at placing needles in direct contact with specific nerves.

Since the skin in most areas of the body is amply supplied with nerves, it is almost impossible to insert a needle anywhere without proximation to pain, touch, and pressure receptors. People with intact nervous systems will , of course, feel the prick when an acupuncture needle is inserted, but the skilled acupuncturist will make needle insertion as painless as possible.

The student of acupuncture must understand that the energy meridian system on which acupuncture points are located is different from the nervous system. The meridians can be thought of as the main channels of energy flow but not as major nerve pathways. The fact that no body energy system is found in cadavers does not mean that it does not exist in the living body. Like other electricity, it is invisible.

DIFFERENCES IN CRITERIA

Because of profound differences between Chinese and Western concepts of etiology, diagnostic procedures, nomenclature, and classification of disease, it is difficult to integrate the two systems of medical practice. Acupuncture was developed before microscopes, X-rays, electrocardiographs, and equipment for biochemical analysis were available. Even in current Chinese periodicals, very little is written about microscopic organisms as etiologic factors, specific metabolic disorders, or electric diagnostic equipment. Instead, the acupuncturist makes a "pulse diagnosis" using criteria which seem irrational to Western scientists.

DIAGNOSES

Since Chinese pulse diagnosis takes a long time to learn, is questionably scientific, and since there are many other good diagnostic procedures available, it seems pointless to teach it to Americans. It is important, however, that an accurate diagnosis, using the best modern methods available, be made before acupuncture treatment is attempted, except for emergency pain relief after injuries. If there is a standard American treatment which is known to be safe and effective for the patient's disorder, he should be given that treatment instead of acupuncture. In general, infections, parasitic infestations, blood dyscracias, tumors, metabolic disorders, and fractures should not be treated by acupuncture, except to relieve pain after its cause has been diagnosed and the patient has had, or is having, standard American treatment. Gout, for instance, is a metabolic disease for which a patient should continue regular treatment while he has acupuncture to relieve arthritic complications. Pain from terminal cancer can be relieved by acupuncture, but acupuncture should not be attempted as a treatment for cancer. We should never take a chance on masking symptoms or delaying potentially curative treatment.

The best uses for acupuncture in the United States are for analgesia and treatment of thoroughly diagnosed, chronic disorders for which there is no other safe treatment or for which drugs or surgery have been tried unsuccessfully. Another possible use of acupuncture is for the relief of severe pain from injuries when giving drugs for pain relief might be dangerous. Gerald L. Looney, M.D., in the Department of Emergency Medicine, Los Angeles County USC Medical Center in California, advocates acupuncture for emergency pain relief instead of analgesic drugs which might alter the patient's level of consciousness and cause serious adverse reactions.

WHICH POINTS TO USE

Although each acupuncturist may eventually develop his own formula for the points to use in treating specific disorders, he should first learn the standard and special points listed in Chapters 2 and 3 and in Part 2. The angle and depth of needle insertion, advisability of electrical potentiation, and length of time the needle should be left in place are decisions each acupuncturist will make on the basis of his evaluation of the patient before each treatment, his reading, his instruction from masters of the art, his own experience, and his knowledge of what structures lie under and nearby the acupuncture points.

ANATOMY AND PHYSIOLOGY

A detailed knowledge of anatomy and physiology is necessary to be a competent acupuncturist, as mentioned in Chapter 1. Whenever an acupuncturist inserts a needle, he should have a mental picture of the structures he is piercing intentionally and which nearby structures he must avoid. Most acupuncture manikins and charts show only superficial landmarks and bones. Anyone attempting acupuncture should be aware of which nerves, blood vessels. and other important structures are in the area he selects for needle insertion. It is possible, however, for technicians to learn how to give acupuncture anesthesia for special procedures, such as dental extractions or normal childbirth, without extensive medical training.

ASEPTIC TECHNIQUES

The same aseptic techniques as used for hypodermic needles should be used for acupuncture needles. Merely soaking the needles in alcohol or boiling them in water is not adequate. Ideally, disposable needles should be used, but standard autoclaving or dry heat of 350°F for 30 minutes destroys viruses and spores as well as bacteria. Wearing disposable gloves is a safe procedure, especially for the beginner who is more likely than the master to touch the shaft of the needle during insertion. Most classical experienced acupuncturists, however, consider gloves a cumbersome and unnecessary inconvenience. It is imperative to avoid introducing the hepatitis virus or other infectious agents into a patient's body.

MOXIBUSTION

The ancient art of moxibustion is still used by the "barefoot doctors" of China, especially in areas where electricity is not yet readily available. Moxibustion is the application of heat to acupuncture points by burning various forms of the herb *artemesia vulgaris* (*Moxi* or *Ai*) over them. This herb burns at a low uniform temperature and some have attributed benefits to its aroma. Research on 3,000 patients comparing moxibustion with infrared light for potentiating the effect of acupuncture at the Washington Acupuncture Center in 1973, however, indicated that infrared light was equally effective, as safe, and esthetically more pleasing to Americans. Therefore, it does not seem important to teach the art of moxibustion here since electricity and infrared lamps are readily available.

ASSOCIATION WITH ORIENTAL HERBOLOGY

In China and other Oriental countries, acupuncture has traditionally been taught in close association with herbology. Most acupuncturists are also herbologists. They are disappointed that the herbs they value most highly are unobtainable in the United States, except in the Chinatowns of a few large cities. Some Oriental herbs, however, are available in American health food stores.

Some of the most useful drugs in the United States, such as digitalis and quinine, have been derived from herbs. Eventually, an effective drug to control bleeding will probably be derived from another Oriental herb. Unfortunately, however, the chemical formula for the effective components of most Oriental herbs has not been determined. The quantity of these components in available preparations has too much variation to meet United States pharmacological standards.

Oriental herbs, such as ginseng, which are available in American health food stores are likely to be contaminated with various substances. These are usually unspecified and may be hazardous.

It may be necessary for a physician supervising Oriental acupuncturists to explain to them that prescribing or dispensing herbs in a medical office constitutes practicing medicine and is prohibited to them. Besides giving patients Oriental herbs, some Oriental acupuncturists may apply ointments with a pungent aroma to the patient's skin. These chemically unanalyzed ointments may cause allergic reactions and have no place in an American medical practice.

SELF-PRACTICE

The most difficult problem in teaching acupuncture to Americans is to convince them that they must practice inserting needles into their own bodies before they are ready to practice on patients. This is essential because there is no other way to learn when and how one has produced the sensation of "energization" (Te-Chi). The manner in which a needle is inserted may determine whether it will stimulate or sedate a certain part of the body or what part of the body will be affected by it. The sensation produced by each insertion is somewhat different. To be aware of the many varieties and locations of sensations resulting from different types of needle insertion, the acupuncturist must learn how to produce these by inserting needles into himself. For instance, a needle inserted perpendicularly into the body on an acupuncture point might cause a sensation of heat in some remote part of the body; insertion of the needle obliquely at the same point might produce instantaneous relief of pain in another part of the body. We have not yet discovered any other way for a student to learn this art.

In order to be a skillful acupuncturist, one must always be conscious of the similarity of the patient's body and feelings to his own. An acupuncturist has to identify closely with the patient and be very conscious of the patient's feelings.

This orientation to medical practice is quite a contrast to that of the American physician who is taught to regard his patient objectively. He is discouraged from prescribing drugs for himself and may accept the slogan "Don't try to be your own doctor." The acupuncturist, on the other hand, must learn to be his own doctor before he is considered fit to be anyone else's doctor. Callous objectivity is abhorrent to acupuncturists.

SPECIALIZATION

Highly skilled acupuncturists do not limit themselves to treating only one part of the body or specialize in certain diseases. The Chinese theories on which acupuncture is based are concerned with the body as a whole and the influence of one part of it on other parts. The Chinese believe that American physicians are very foolish to compartmentalize medical practice. They think that any physician who limits his medical practice to any specialty may miss the correct diagnosis and is likely to prescribe treatment that might temporarily relieve symptoms in one area while injuring other areas and the body as a whole. Acupuncture treatment is intended to restore the balance of positive and negative body energy (*Yang* and *Yin*) and thereby improve a person's general health as well as relieving pain or malfunction in specific parts of the body.

A physician should be able to learn the basic techniques of acupuncture in about 400 hours, enough to give lasting pain relief to many patients without giving them drugs. Anesthesiologists, dentists, and paramedics could learn how to give acupuncture analgesia for specific procedures or to relieve pain temporarily with even less training. Safe acupuncture should soon be an alternative available to anyone who needs pain relief without risking adverse drug reactions.

In contrast to the United States where the most highly trained physicians are usually specialists, acupuncturists who specialize in giving acupuncture analgesia for specific procedures or to relieve pain in certain parts of the body are the ones with the least training. Giving effective acupuncture to restore function to nerve tissues, to treat allergic, psychiatric, or other systemic disorders usually takes years of training and experience.

chapter 7

DETERMINING WHETHER ACUPUNCTURE IS THE TREATMENT OF CHOICE

Determining whether acupuncture is the treatment of choice depends on the availability, as well as the relative safety and effectiveness, of alternative treatments. For this reason, it is essential that the physician who examines a patient be aware of, and utilize, appropriate diagnostic procedures and treatments other than acupuncture, as needed. Acupuncture should never be used to mask symptoms or to delay proper medical treatment. An acupuncturist who does not know the English language and has had no medical training in the United

States should not be given the responsibility of deciding whether acupuncture is the treatment of choice. On the other hand, in an emergency situation, acupuncture is much safer than drugs for relieving pain before definitive diagnosis and treatment are available. It is less likely than analgesic drugs to alter the patient's level of consciousness, mask symptoms, or create allergic reactions and other undesirable side effects.

ALTERNATIVES

As mentioned in previous chapters, acupuncture in the United States is used mainly for the treatment of chronic disorders and analgesia. Although it is sometimes a valuable adjunct to conventional treatment, it should not be used as a substitute for antibiotics, chemotherapy, nutritional therapy, or other specific treatment modalities. In disorders for which drugs and/or surgical procedures are available but hazardous or damaging to general health, acupuncture should be considered. The cortisone derivatives, gold salts, and phenylbutazone routinely prescribed for arthritis, for instance, can have lethal side effects and at best relieve symptoms temporarily. Surgery for arthritis may make the condition worse; lasting good results are rare. Acupuncture gives no undesirable side effects and may be more effective than drugs or surgery for most cases of arthritis.

RELATIVE EXPENSE

Although the relative expense of available treatments should not be a factor in determining the type of treatment a patient receives, it often is. Acupuncture is the least expensive, as well as the safest and most effective, treatment for many chronic disorders. It can usually be given on an outpatient basis. Patients who have acupuncture anesthesia for surgery usually recover more rapidly and can leave the hospital sooner than those who have had chemical anesthesia. In some cases, acupuncture can enable people crippled with arthritis or neurological disorders to become self-sufficient enough to get along without nursing care. Some patients, as well as their relatives and friends, can even be taught to give enough acupuncture or acupressure to relieve a specific type of pain without the danger or expense of drugs.

PATIENT'S MEDICAL HISTORY

Before acupuncture treatment is recommended, a detailed medical history should be obtained to rule out all of the conditions for which alternative treatment might be more effective. If such a condition is discovered or suspected, the patient should, of course, be referred to an appropriate specialist or clinic.

A patient should be questioned about his diet and vitamin intake to rule out nutritional problems. He should also be questioned about exposure to toxic substances in his environment and the drugs which he has been taking. Unfortunately, many patients do not know the names of the drugs they are taking and will deny that they have been warned about possible side effects. When asked to bring their drugs to the office for identification, many of them bring a shopping bag full of prescription bottles.

In some cases it will be found that drugs are causing or aggravating symptoms. Patients taking cortisone or its derivatives, for instance, may have signs of subcutaneous bleeding, moon fauces, and/or other disorders masked by the drug. Patients taking major tranquilizers may have symptoms of dyskinesia and other neurologic problems.

It is important to know which drugs can safely be discontinued abruptly and which must be tapered off gradually to avoid serious withdrawal symptoms. Some drugs, of course, must be continued indefinitely, both during and after acupuncture treatments. Failure to discuss medications with a patient can lead to serious problems during acupuncture therapy.

PROHIBITIONS

Although each patient must be evaluated individually, there are many medical conditions for which acupuncture is not the treatment of choice in the United States. Acupuncture is not harmful to people with the medical problems listed below but it might relieve symptoms sufficiently to cause a delay in obtaining other more specific treatment. People with heart disease, for instance, can have their arthritis or other medical problems treated by acupuncture, but should not expect acupuncture to be a substitute for such treatment as digitalis, oxygen, nutritional therapy, and carefully monitored exercise. Since acupuncture can promote abortion, the Washington Acupuncture Center has refused to treat pregnant women. The following list is a guideline for conditions not to be treated by acupuncture. This list is not all-inclusive.

CONDITIONS NOT TO BE TREATED BY ACUPUNCTURE

1. Infections.
2. Parasitic infestations.
3. Blood and blood vessel abnormalities (except to stimulate circulation to ischemic areas, as in Raynaud's or Buerger's disease).
4. Heart disease.
5. Neoplasms.
6. Urinary tract diseases, such as nephritis, nephrosis, or cystitis.
7. Metabolic diseases, such as diabetes, thyroid problems, hypoglycemia, or malnutrition.
8. Pregnancy (except for initiation of labor or as analgesia for delivery).
9. Vaginal discharges.
10. Prostate disorders.
11. Otosclerosis and other middle ear abnormalities.
12. Emphysema (except for allergic symptoms associated with it).
13. Eye problems (except neurogenic blindness or manifestations of multiple sclerosis).
14. Fractures.
15. Acute surgical conditions, such as appendicitis or ruptured viscera.
16. Severed nerves.

DIAGNOSTIC USE

Acupuncture can be used safely in place of some painful diagnostic procedures. For instance, in cases of lumbar disc pathology, it is generally safer to attempt to relieve symptoms with acupuncture than to perform a myelogram for diagnostic purposes. If the orthopedic problem is serious enough to require laminectomy, acupuncture will not give lasting relief of symptoms. In this sense, acupuncture might be considered a safer and less painful diagnostic procedure than a myelogram. The latter must be used when surgery is contemplated.

Most headaches respond well to acupuncture therapy, but before recommending acupuncture, the physician should make sure the headache is not caused by a brain tumor, aneurysm, or arteritis. If a patient has had the same type of headache periodically for a number of years, diagnostic procedures such as electroencephalograms, tomography, and skull X-rays will usually have been performed before he seeks acupuncture. It is generally unnecessary to repeat diagnostic procedures before acupuncture treatment is given for such headaches unless there has been some significant change in the patient's symptoms.

Since acupuncture was considered a complete system of medical practice by the ancient Chinese, most of the books on traditional acupuncture prescribe this treatment procedure for conditions for which it should not be used in the United States. These Oriental books also give concepts of etiology, diagnostic criteria and nomenclature which are difficult to translate into language meaningful to Americans. In spite of such problems, these books contain valuable information which can be integrated with modern medical practice. Ignoring the excellent diagnostic procedures and scientific knowledge available in the United States, however, would be a serious mistake.

COMBINATION WITH NUTRITIONAL THERAPY

Most patients seeking acupuncture treatments have had their nutritional status impaired by drugs which have been prescribed for their ailments. Taking vitamin and mineral supplements for optimal nutrition enables them to obtain maximal benefit from acupuncture treatments.

Like acupuncture, nutritional therapy is generally a safe way to treat chronic physical and mental disorders. It has become almost impossible to obtain a nutritionally adequate diet free from undesirable contaminants in the United States. The "minimal daily requirements" are inadequate for counteracting damage to health from disease, drugs, and pollutants in food, water, and air.

Each person has different nutritional requirements depending on his personal physiology and environmental conditions. Unfortunately, most physicians have not been trained to determine what these requirements are and seem reluctant to provide nutritional therapy along with other treatment modalities. Many physicians prescribe drugs which greatly increase a patient's need for certain vitamins or minerals but neglect to inform him about this. Each patient should discuss his individual requirements with his physician.

Although huge overdoses of some vitamins may be dangerous, and high doses of certain B vitamins may cause excessive excretion of other B vitamins, thereby resulting in deficiencies, most vitamins are non-toxic to most people. The Washington Acupuncture Center physicians usually recommend that patients supplement their diet with at least the following vitamins and minerals daily. Most of these are available in combinations to reduce the number of pills or capsules required to obtain optimal daily doses.

DAILY VITAMIN AND MINERAL SUPPLEMENTS

Vitamin A	10,000 I.U.*	Calcium	200 mg
Vitamin B$_1$	(Thiamin) 20 mg	Magnesium	60 mg.
Vitamin B$_2$	(Riboflavin) 20 mg.	Zinc	30 mg.
Vitamin B$_6$	(Pyridoxine) 20 mg.		
Vitamin B$_{12}$	50 mcg.		
Niacinamide	500 mg.		
Folic acid	.1 mg.		
Biotin	20 mcg.		
Choline	20 mg.		
Inositol	20 mg.		
PABA (para-amino-benzoic acid)	10 mg.		
Pantothenic acid	50 mg.		
Vitamin C (ascorbic acid)	1000 mg.		
Vitamin D	400 I.U.*		
Vitamin E	100 I.U.*		

*International Units.

The above listed quantities of vitamins and minerals can be taken daily without any danger of toxicity. Pure vitamins are not allergenic. However, some vitamin preparations contain yeast and/or rose "hips," which may be allergenic. It is possible to obtain preparations of vitamins and minerals free of these substances. Anyone experiencing an apparent allergic reaction to vitamin or mineral preparations should discuss this problem with his physician.

Continuing nutritional therapy after completion of acupuncture treatments increases the likelihood that the results of acupuncture will be lasting. The quantities of vitamin and mineral supplements an individual needs for optimal health should be reevaluated at least every six months. Dietary changes should also be considered as weight approaches normal and the patient is able to lead a more active life, free from the restrictions of pain and disabilities.

COMBINATION WITH OTHER TREATMENTS

One of the advantages of acupuncture is that it does not interfere with other treatments. It can be used to relieve the pain of cancer while the patient is receiving chemotherapy or other treatments. It can also be used to reduce the seizures of epilepsy while patients continue to take anticonvulsant drugs. People being treated for heart disease, diabetes, or other conditions for which acupuncture is not the treatment of choice can, at the same time, have acupuncture treatments for their arthritis or other disorders for which acupuncture is appropriate. Many elderly or highly allergic patients who are unable to tolerate analgesic drugs or surgery can have pain safely relieved by acupuncture. This treatment can be used instead of psychotropic drugs to relieve anxiety, insomnia, depression, and hyperactivity while a patient is given psychotherapy.

AFTER OTHER TREATMENT HAS FAILED

Acupuncture has been found very successful for treating sexual impotence in cases where organic pathology has been ruled out. Some patients who have not responded to months of psychotherapy for this problem have had their potency restored after six to ten acupuncture treatments. There is no reason, however, to discontinue psychotherapy during the time a patient is being treated with acupuncture.

Although there is still no satisfactory explanation of how or why acupuncture can be therapeutic for paresis, it often gives relief of symptoms in neurologic disorders and other ailments for which no other treatment is available. Before a patient is told that he has no hope of improvement in his condition, he should be given a chance to have acupuncture treatments. Many patients with diseases described as untreatable, or progressive without remission, have experienced significant improvement through acupuncture.

chapter 8

TECHNIQUES AND PRECAUTIONS

The techniques used for acupuncture treatment are in many ways similar to those for giving other medical treatments. Each acupuncturist will tend to develop his own style of needle insertion but should always be concerned about asepsis and the physical and emotional welfare of his patients.

ENVIRONMENT AND POSITION

The environment for giving acupuncture treatment should be a room in a physician's office which is equipped for minor surgery. However, acupuncture can be administered in a patient's bedroom, an ambulance, or elsewhere. In most cases, the patient should recline on an examining or treatment table, although it is sometimes desirable to treat patients in a sitting position. It is important that the position selected for each treatment be comfortable to the patient and that he be encouraged to relax before, during, and after the treatment to maximize the benefit he will derive from it. Some acupuncturists ask their patients to recline on the treatment table for as long as half an hour before treatment begins.

ASEPSIS

Prior to sterilization, all needles and other equipment should be checked carefully. Needles should be sharp, clean, straight, and not have loose handles. All equipment should be autoclaved or heated dry at 350°F for at least 30 minutes to destroy all bacteria, viruses, and spores. After sterilization, the needles should not be touched or contaminated in any way before insertion. Skin areas surrounding the acupuncture points to be used should be cleansed with alcohol or Zephiran. Acupuncturists should wear sterile disposable gloves or at least scrub their hands with antiseptic soap.

DEPTH OF NEEDLE INSERTION

The depth of needle insertion depends on the anatomical location of the acupuncture point and the vitality of the patient. Most acupuncture points are located in the corium, the connective tissue layer beneath the dermis of the skin. Chinese medical books, however, describe some acupuncture points as being in the spaces between muscles, tendons and bones.

Experienced acupuncturists can sense the achievement of *Te-Chi* by the pressure of local muscle contraction exerted around the needle, as if slight suction were applied to the tip of the needle. This phenomenon indicates that the needle has reached the appropriate depth. The skin coloration produced by vasodilation can be another sign indicating the extent of somatosensory stimulation. The acupuncturist should pay special attention to the patient's local responses and sensations during needle insertion. If the patient does not feel *Te-Chi* when the needle is inserted to the prescribed depth, the needle should be withdrawn and electric point-finding instruments should be used for more precise point location.

Very few acupuncture points require needle insertions deeper than one-half *cun* (5 *fen*). The most commonly used acupuncture point which requires a long needle and deep insertion (1.5–3 *cun*, depending on the size and shape of the patient's body) is GB 30 (Huantiao), located near the hip joint. Branches of gluteal nerves and the sciatic nerve converge in this region. The major femoral artery and vein pass underneath the femoral joint and should, of course, be avoided. Acupuncture point GB 30 is used for treating sciatica, arthritis, leg paralysis, multiple sclerosis, and muscle spasm, some of the conditions most frequently treated by acupuncture.

There are a few other acupuncture points which require relatively deep needle insertion (1.0–1.5 *cun*). The most frequently used ones are: Co 10 and 11, St 31, and GB 31. These four acupuncture points are used for treating arthritis, neurological diseases, and muscular malfunctions. Co 11 is a very important point used in the treatment of arthritis and skin problems.

As a general rule, all needle insertions on the head, neck and chest should be superficial—only a few millimeters in depth. The eyes and eardrums should be carefully avoided. In the neck, the carotid arteries, jugular veins, and other blood vessels are very superficial in some patients, especially in the old and debilitated.

The depths of insertion for the thoracic region should be shallow. Needles in this area should not be twirled or manipulated except by highly skilled acupuncturists in unusually resistant cases. Pneumothorax may result if the pleura and lungs are accidentally punctured. Serious bleeding may result if major arteries and veins or visceral organs are damaged. Safety of the patient should be the first consideration.

DANGEROUS AREAS

There are some important areas close to vital organs and blood vessels where acupuncture treatment should be avoided. These are:

1. The "triangle of auscultation" between the scapulae.
2. The axillary area where the axillary artery and vein are quite superficial.
3. Over the heart.
4. The upper anterior chest.
5. Over the brain, in patients with skull defects.
6. Over the urinary bladder in the lower abdomen.
7. Over the kidneys, on the back.
8. Over the mammary arteries, within 2–4 cm. of the sternum.

Generally speaking, needle insertion near the viscera or arteries must be carefully avoided. Any points used for treatment in these areas require superficial insertion and the expertise of a highly skilled acupuncturist with a thorough knowledge of anatomy. The beginning acupuncturist should refrain from inserting needles in or near the sex organs, eyes, ear drums, and nipples.

FORBIDDEN POINTS OF ACUPUNCTURE

Many forbidden points are described in Chinese medical books. Due to current medical developments and experimentation, some points are no longer considered forbidden. The forbidden points are usually located near major arteries, veins, and visceral structures. They include the following:

Forbidden points

Brain 10, 11, 17, 22, and 24

Gall Bladder 18

Heart 2

Kidney 11

Liver 10 and 12

Metabolism 8, 19, and 20

Sex 1, 9, 17, and 18

Spleen 11

Stomach 17 and 30

Urinary Bladder 9 and 56

Forbidden points for pregnant women
(except for delivery)

Colon 4

Spleen 12

Stomach 12 and all points on the abdomen.

EMERGENCIES DURING TREATMENT

Since acupuncture is a relatively safe procedure, few emergencies are likely to arise during therapy. Needles should be of good quality and inspected before sterilization to avoid the possibility of a broken needle. Patients should be asked to lie still to avoid bending the needles. If a patient does become restless, needles should be removed promptly. If patients are in a reclining position, syncope is unlikely. Seizures on the treatment table should be treated as seizures elsewhere, except that the needles should be removed promptly.

If an acupuncture needle should break with a portion left in the patient, the acupuncturist should instruct the patient to remain motionless. If the broken needle remains visible outside the body, the acupuncturist can slowly remove the needle with a pair of tweezers. If the broken needle has been buried under the skin, X-ray examination and surgical removal may be necessary. The use of high quality stainless steel needles makes needle breakage extremely unlikely.

If the patient suddenly becomes pale, sweats profusely, appears nervous, feels dizzy or nauseated, he may be suffering from hypotension, decreased cerebral circulation, or hypoxia. Probably the most common cause is a vaso-vagal syncopal reaction. Other causes of syncope include hypoglycemia, diabetic hyperglycemic coma, adrenal crisis from cortisone withdrawal, pneumothorax, cerebral vascular occlusion or hemorrhage, cardiac tamponade, pulmonary embolism, and vascular collapse secondary to myocardial insufficiency.

If any of the foregoing complications arise, acupuncture needles should be withdrawn immediately. The patient should be lying down comfortably and have his legs elevated a little. Blood pressure, pulse rate, and respiratory rate should be obtained at once. Patency of the airway should be determined and oxygen administered, if indicated, under constant supervision. Standard emergency diagnostic and treatment procedures should be instituted promptly.

It is important to explain acupuncture procedures and related details to the patient before treatment and to answer his questions. An adequate pretreatment history regarding current medication and past syncopal episodes, seizures, or abnormalities of the cardiovascular system is essential. This information may greatly facilitate the diagnosis and treatment of an apparent syncopal episode.

Bleeding, external or internal, is seldom a problem with acupuncture, because the needles are thin and inserted superficially, away from blood vessels. Patients who have been taking cortisone, aspirin, anticoagulants, various other drugs, or unusually large doses of Vitamin E, however, tend to bleed easily. Many subcutaneous bruises may be evident as a warning and should be avoided by acupuncture needles. If the acupuncturist should accidentally pierce a blood vessel and produce external or internal bleeding with swelling and discoloration, the area should be elevated above the heart if possible and external pressure applied with sterile gauze over the bleeding area. Appropriate pressure points for stopping hemorrhage may also be used. Ice packs may reduce pain and swelling. Massage of the area may cause an increase in subcutaneous bleeding or thromboembolic phenomena and should not be attempted. It is extremely unusual, however, for a patient to lose more than one or two drops of blood during acupuncture treatment.

NEEDLE TECHNIQUE

Beginning acupuncturists should use short needles of high quality with shafts less than an inch long to avoid inserting them too deeply. Gold is too soft and silver too corrosive to be used for acupuncture needles.

By the time an acupuncturist inserts needles into other people, he should have practiced enough on himself to have skill in making needle insertion as painless and accurate as possible. The needles should be adjusted gently to give the patient the *Te-Chi* sensation. They may be twirled for stimulation but generally are left in place for about twenty minutes and then removed. Acupuncture should be a bloodless and almost painless procedure.

Techniques for electric and heat potentiation of acupuncture needles are described in Chapter 9.

ELECTRO-ACUPUNCTURE

Electro-acupuncture is acupuncture using electricity for point-finding and/or potentiation.

RELATION TO TRANSCUTANEOUS ELECTRIC STIMULATION

When electro-acupuncture is used for potentiation, it may be called percutaneous or transcutaneous electric stimulation (TES). TES is sometimes performed with electrodes which do not penetrate the skin and is thus similar to electro-acupressure. Most people who use TES are trying to stimulate a specific nerve or nerve plexus rather than acupuncture points, whether they insert needles through the skin or not. Many acupuncture points are located over nerve fibers, but acupuncturists are not trying to pierce nerve fibers. Although acupuncture without electric potentiation, TES without piercing the skin, TES piercing the skin, and electro-acupressure can all stimulate the body to produce endorphins (endogenous morphine-like biochemicals discussed in Chapter 5), electro-acupuncture by skilled acupuncturists is the most effective technique for this purpose.[1,2]

HISTORY

Louis Berlioz,[3] a French physician, first reported the potentiating effects of electro-acupuncture in 1816. In 1825, another French physician, Sarlandiere,[4] reported the use of this technique for the treatment of gout, rheumatism, and other ailments. Sarlandiere connected a metal conducting wire to an acupuncture needle after the needle had been inserted into the body. A glass tube was placed over the external portion of the needle to insulate it and a switch was used to control the flow of electricity. In 1832, F.W. Becker,[5] a German, published an article on "Galvanopunctur" in *Medicinische Zeitung.* Electro-acupuncture was used as anesthesia for removal of a "glandular tumor" in the United States by L.H. Cohen in 1875.[6]

Since 1955, instruments have been designed which can be used for both point location and therapy. They indicate that resistance is lower and electric potential higher at acupuncture points than on adjacent areas of the skin.[7] These instruments can be adjusted to use a direct or pulsating current for augmentation of acupuncture.[8] Many instruments of this type are now being used by acupuncturists in America and elsewhere.[9]

Although electro-acupuncture was practiced at different times by Chinese and other Oriental people, those who practiced it did not write much about it until the middle of this century. Since then it has been used by most of the acupuncturists in China, including the "barefoot doctors."[10]

NEUROPHYSIOLOGIC PROBLEMS

From a physical and physiologic viewpoint, the needle supplies a mechanical stimulus which is augmented by the electricity. It is not clearly understood why the stimulation must be made at particular points in order to achieve the desired effects.

Early electro-acupuncture practitioners used induced current to demonstrate that acupuncture points have low resistance to electricity and therefore permit a larger flow of electric current to pass through them. Research on the implications of this observation has continued,[11] but theories linking positively charged acupuncture points and organs with *Yang*, and negatively charged points with *Yin*, have not been supported by scientific data.

EQUIPMENT AND METHODS OF APPLICATION

The basic principles of electro-acupuncture instruments are the same, regardless of the model (Fig. 9–1). The source of power can be derived from a battery or from a wall socket. A vibrating mechanism which includes switches and potentiometers is required to control the frequencies and wave forms of the current. A controlling apparatus is needed to regulate the strength of the electric current. The power supply of an electro-acupuncture instrument is generally 3 to 6 volts. When using wall-socket electricity, it is necessary to use a transformer to reduce the voltage.

The function of the vibrator is to cause the electric current to vibrate at a certain frequency, with a specific type of wave form. The frequency should be at least 10–200 per minute. There are different types of waves, i.e., sawtooth, pulsating, square, sine, etc. Square and sine waves should not be used for acupuncture potentiation. The pulsating waves are used most frequently. Improper types of waves can be painful and/or ineffective.

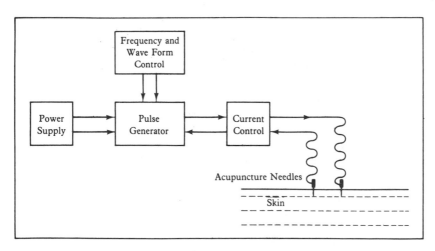

Figure 9–1.   Block diagram of basic instrument for electric potentiation of acupuncture

After two acupuncture needles are inserted in the skin, electrodes from the instrument are tightly clasped to the handles of the needles. The body fluids and tissues between the two needles complete the circuit for the electric current. To avoid excess electric current, the instrument should be designed to produce only a minimal amount of current. Generally, 25–200 microamperes are sufficient to achieve the desired effect.

The electric current is thought to produce various complex biochemical and physical changes. These changes depend on the nature and strength of the electricity as well as on the choice of acupuncture points. Those who undergo electro-acupuncture treatment generally experience paresthesia, a feeling of heaviness or mild aching, but the electric current should not be painful. For the treatment of most medical problems, the electro-acupuncture instruments are attached for 20 minutes.

There are many types of electro-acupuncture instruments now in use. The following are some which have been in clinical use for more than 30 years:

1.   Battery-operated direct current.

2.   Induction.

3.   Alternating current converted to pulsating current.

4.   Electronic vibrating.

5.   Semiconductor.

A purely direct electric current has a very strong sedating effect. In the application of direct current electro-acupuncture, however, electrolysis may occur if the needle is made of two different metals. In order to prevent electrolysis, it is necessary to keep the electric poles alternating. Although the sedating effect of the pulsating current is slightly below that of the purely direct current, electrolysis is not likely to occur. When it is necessary to have a comparatively stronger sedating effect, the flow of current can be prolonged and a weaker current used.

The stimulating effect is greater with induced electric current than with pulsating currents, but the sedating effect is less. When induced electric current is used in electro-acupuncture, it often produces a strong contraction of muscles. Careful medical evaluation of the patient is, therefore, essential before it is used. The stimulating effect is not as strong in pulsating currents, but in general use it is quite satisfactory. A pulsating current with a sawtooth wave is usually used for acupuncture anesthesia.

Electronic and semiconductor types of electro-acupuncture instruments are somewhat similar to pulsating current instruments, having both sedating and stimulating functions. The wave type produced by these instruments must be exact. Acupuncture instruments should be tested regularly with an oscilloscope to be sure that they are delivering the correct type of wave.

The majority of illnesses do not need strong sedation or stimulation. The length of time that electricity is used and the strength and type of current desired influence the decision as to which type of instrument to use.

ELECTRO-ACUPUNCTURE ANESTHESIA OR ANALGESIA

To maintain adequate levels of acupuncture for surgery, electric potentiation of the needles is usually required throughout the procedure. Induction of anesthesia generally takes about 20 minutes. Anesthesia can be maintained for prolonged periods of time as long as the electro-acupuncture instruments are connected to the needles. A pulsating current instrument set for a sawtooth wave is generally the most satisfactory for this purpose. The strength of the current varies depending on the patient's sensitivity to it. Usually 50–200 microamperes give satisfactory results. This subject is discussed further in Chapter 13.

HEAT LAMP POTENTIATION

Infrared rays produce a penetrating warm sensation which may potentiate the needle alone or with electro-acupuncture. The Washington Acupuncture Center uses infrared rays as a substitute for moxibustion. After two years of experimentation (1973–75), it seemed evident that infrared heat was as effective for potentiation as burning *moxa* over the acupuncture points. Many patients had complained about the marijuana-like aroma of moxibustion as well as the danger of being burned by it.

An infrared ray lamp of 100–200 watts can be directed at a group of meridian points. White cardboard can be used to cover the area around the points, but this is usually unnecessary. The source of light should be approximately 18–24 inches away from the skin. The lamp may be regulated to produce a sensation of warmth, without burning the skin.

VALUE OF ELECTRO-ACUPUNCTURE

Electric point-locating systems diminish the possibility of selecting the wrong sites for needle insertion. The various techniques of electro-acupuncture may reduce the time required for acupuncture treatment and the number of treatments required to achieve therapeutic results. Electro-acupuncture eliminates the necessity of handtwirling needles for potentiation. Although highly skilled acupuncturists seldom use electric point-locating instruments and can produce adequate analgesia for surgery without electric potentiation, most acupuncturists find electro-acupuncture instruments useful for treatment, analgesia, and research.

REFERENCES FOR CHAPTER 9

1. Fox, J. Elisabeth; and Melzak, Ronald. "Transcutaneous Electric Stimulation and Acupuncture." *Pain* 2 (Amsterdam 1976): 141–148.

2. Sjölund, Bengt; and Eriksson, Margareta. "Electro-Acupuncture and Endogenous Morphines." *Lancet* 2 (November 1976): 1085.

3. Berlioz, Louis. *Memories Sur les Maladie Chronique, les Evacuations Sanguines et l'Acupuncture.* Paris: Croullebois, 1816 (343 pp.).

4. Sarlandiere, Jean Baptiste. *Memoires sur l'Ectro-puncture, Considerée Comme Moyen Nouveau de Traiter Efficacement la Goute, les Rhumatismes et les Affections Nerveuses.* Paris, 1825 (150 pp.).

5. Becker, F.W. "Über die Wirkungen der Galvanopunctur." *Medicinishe Zeitung* 6 (October 10, 1832): 23–25.

6. Cohen, L.H. "Galvanopuncture; with a Successful Case of Operation by Electrolysis in a Glandular Tumor." *New York Medical Journal* 22 (1875): 380–387.

7. Bergsman, O.; and Wooley-Hart, A. "Differences in Electrical Skin Conductivity between Acupuncture Points and Adjacent Skin Areas." *American Journal of Acupuncture* 1 (1973): 27–32.

8. Lee, S.K. "The Application and Construction of Electro-Acu-

puncture Apparatus." *Fukien Journal of Chinese Medicine,* September 1958.

9. Voll, R. "Twenty Years of Electroacupuncture Therapy Using Low Frequency Current Pulses." *American Journal of Acupuncture* 3 (1975): 291–314.

10. Silverstein, Martin E.; Chang, I-Lok; and Mason, Nathaniel (translators) *Acupuncture and Moxibustion, A Handbook for the Barefoot Doctors of China.* New York: Schocken Books, 1975.

11. Becker, R.O.; Reichmanis, M.; Marino, A.A.; and Spadaro, J.A. "Electrophysiological Correlates of Acupuncture Points and Meridians." *Psychoenergetic Systems* 1 (1976): 105–114.

chapter 10

CLINICAL RESEARCH

As discussed in Chapter 5, basic research to determine the neurophysiologic mechanisms in the effects of acupuncture is being done by biochemists and other physical scientists in many different countries. Considerable progress has been made, especially with regard to endorphins, but many questions remain to be answered.

The skill of acupuncturists participating in both basic and clinical acupuncture research is a very important factor which is difficult for most Americans to evaluate. It is expected that when more Americans gain knowledge of acupuncture, this problem will be minimized. Unless skilled acupuncturists are used for acupuncture research, its results may be invalid.

EVALUATING THE EFFECTIVENESS OF ACUPUNCTURE FOR RELIEVING PAIN

Pain is a subjective symptom which is impossible to measure precisely. Words are inadequate to give an accurate description of pain. Similar physical injuries or disease pathology seem to give different qualities and quantities of pain to different people. Such factors as age, size, sex, skin color, and nationality do not seem to affect the pain a person feels, but cultural conditioning can influence a person's reaction to pain and ability to cope with it without complaining. People who say that Orientals are less sensitive to pain than Caucasians are revealing their racial prejudice rather than knowledge.

Various techniques and devices for measuring pain have been tried, but none has proved entirely satisfactory. What a patient says and does about his pain is still one of the most reliable indicators of the quality and quantity of pain he is feeling. It is difficult to discount the placebo effect and the influence of such emotional factors as fear, anxiety, and depression. No research involving measuring pain or comparing the pain of one person with that of another can be completely objective or scientific. The research done by the Washington Acupuncture Center from 1973 to 1976 to measure the results of acupuncture treatments on people with pain syndromes encountered these problems. The pain relief or "improvement" recorded for each patient was based on what the patient said.

EVALUATING THE EFFECTS ON EMOTIONAL AND BEHAVIORAL DISORDERS

In attempting to quantify changes in depression, insomnia, or sexual potency, one has to depend on interviews and questionnaires, which are not necessarily reliable. Spouses' comments were taken into consideration whenever possible in evaluating the results of acupuncture treatment for these conditions, but such comments might have been motivated by unknown factors. Blood tests were not performed to check for alcohol or drugs.

WEIGHT REDUCTION AND HEARING IMPROVEMENT

Weight reduction was the most objective measurement in evaluating results of acupuncture. Treatments for this problem were usually given on a weekly basis. Patients who lost at least three pounds a week were classified as having "significant improvement." Patients who lost at least one pound but less than three pounds a week were classified as having "slight improvement." Many patients have reported that their greatest weight loss came during the three months after they completed their acupuncture treatments, but these reports were not included in the research data.

Hearing improvement was another objective measurement. Tests for discrimination as well as sound level were given using a sound-proof booth and standardized voice recordings. It was found that almost all patients with neurogenic hearing loss had their discrimination improved by acupuncture but only about half of them experienced more than a fifteen decibel improvement in sound level at four or more different frequencies. Those with only discrimination improvement were classified as "slight" while those who also had at least a fifteen decibel improvement in sound level of hearing were classified as "significant."

MEASURING FUNCTIONAL IMPROVEMENT FOR ACUPUNCTURE

The Washington Acupuncture Center worked out research protocols for evaluating the results of acupuncture as objectively as possible in patients treated for allergies, arthritis, bursitis, multiple sclerosis, paresis, and Parkinsonism. An example of the research protocol used for arthritis is shown in Figure 10–1.

The data accumulated for this research project was voluminous and difficult to assemble for presentation in a meaningful way. It is easy to criticize the lack of objectivity in collecting some of the data.

GENERAL CRITERIA FOR CLINICAL ACUPUNCTURE RESEARCH

The results of clinical research to determine the effectiveness of acupuncture for treating various conditions can be misleading unless all of the patients included have at least six treatments for conditions involving relief of pain, allergies, psychiatric problems, and addictions. Patients included in studies to evaluate the effectiveness of acupuncture for conditions involving impaired function, such as paresis or neurogenic hearing loss, should have at least ten treatments.

Unless skilled acupuncturists are used for clinical research, the results are meaningless. All of the acupuncturists participating in research at the Washington Acupuncture Center had had at least six years of training in acupuncture and at least ten years of experience.

It would be better to have patients evaluated before and after acupuncture treatments by physicians who had no relationship to the clinic where acupuncture was performed.

Instead of trying to evaluate the improvement of a group of heterogeneous patients, it would be better to compare groups of matched

SAMPLE RESEARCH PROTOCOL

Title: EVALUATION OF ACUPUNCTURE TREATMENT FOR ARTHRITIS

Purpose: ANALYSIS OF ARTHRITIS SYMPTOMS OF PATIENTS BEFORE AND
             AFTER ACUPUNCTURE

Methods: All patients with a diagnosis of arthritis will be examined before and after
             completion of acupuncture treatments using the attached survey form.
             M.D.'s who do not give the treatments will perform these examinations.
             Following acupuncture treatments, the degree of patient improvement will
             be estimated using the following criteria. Sedimentation rates and Rheu-
             matoid factor will be measured by George Washington University Micro-
             biology Department.

Research   Yang Ming Chu, Ph.D., George Washington University
Directors: Yao Wu (Sam) Lee, O.M.D., Ph.D., Washington Acupuncture Center
             Daniel Weiner, M.D., Ph.D., Veterans Administration Hospital

Remission Index	Condition of Patient
0	No improvement in severity or frequency of pain and no decrease in use of analgesic medication
1+	25% reduction in use of analgesic medication with or without increased range of motion in involved joints, or increased range of motion with stable pain pattern
2+	50% reduction in use of analgesic medication and/or 50% increase in joint mobility and 50% decrease in anti-inflammatory medication
3+	Complete remission of pain, at least 50% reduction of inflammation, more than 50% increase in range of motion of involved joints
4+	Normal sedimentation rate, complete remission of pain, at least 80% reduc-tion of inflammation, freedom from analgesic and anti-inflammatory medica-tion, at least 80% improvement in range of motion of involved joints

All patients included in this research will have at least six treatments at the Washington
Acupuncture Center. Number of treatments each patient receives will be recorded.

Follow-up examinations will be given each patient at least yearly for three years.

Figure 10–1.

ARTHRITIS SURVEY

Patient Name _____

Age _____

Date of Examination _____

Total duration of symptoms _____

1. Functional Class

_____

| A. Ability to carry out all usual duties without handicaps. | B. Can conduct normal activities despite discomfort or limited mobility of one or more joints. | C. Capacity adequate to perform only a few or none of the duties of usual occupation or self care. | D. Largely or wholly incapacitated with patient bedridden or confined to wheel chair. |

2. JOINTS INVOLVED (specify degree of change)

Spine-Cervical _____   Thoracic _____ Lumbar____ _____

	Right	*Left*
Shoulder	_____	_____
Elbow	_____	_____
Wrist	_____	_____
Hand	_____	_____
Hip	_____	_____
Knee	_____	_____
Ankle	_____	_____
Foot	_____	_____

1. Pain, but no joint deformities, although limitation of joint mobility may be present.
2. Swelling (soft tissue thickening or fluid).
3. Joint deformity, such as subluxation, ulnar deviation, or hyperextension.
4. Fibrous or bony ankylosis.

For Hand

Joint	Right Digit Involved	Left Digit Involved
Metacarpophalangeal	1 2 3 4 5	1 2 3 4 5
Proximal Interphalangeal	1 2 3 4 5	1 2 3 4 5
Distal Interphalangeal	1 2 3 4 5	1 2 3 4 5

3. PAIN

01 Less than 4 aspirin per day
02 More than 4 aspirin per day
03 Medication more potent than aspirin required
04 Pain relief inadequate with analgesic regime used

Figure 10-1. (Cont'd)

4. Systemic Complications

1. Subcutaneous and subperiosteal nodules (rheumatoid granulomas)

2. Organ involvement	
Heart	Pericarditis, only occasionally sympto-matic and only rarely progressing to chronic constricting disease
	Cardiomyopathy, with conduction defects, resulting from rheumatoid granulomas in myocardium
	Valvular lesions, chiefly aortic, due to rheu-matoid granulomas (rare)
Lung	Pleurisy, with or without effusion
	Multiple pulmonary (rheumatoid) nodules
	Rheumatoid pneumoconiosis (Caplan's syndrome)
	Progressive interstitial fibrosis, with forma-tion of "honeycomb" lung
	Pulmonary arteritis with pulmonary hyper-tension (rare)
Eye	Scleritis, rarely complicated by scleromalacia perforans
	Iridocyclitis
Nervous System	Rheumatoid granulomas in dura mater
	Peripheral neuropathy
	Peripheral compression syndromes, including carpal tunnel syndrome (median neuropathy), ulnar neuropathy, peroneal palsy

3. Systematic complications

    Anemia
    Generalized osteoporosis
    Felty's Syndrome
    Sjögren's syndrome (keratoconjunctivitis sicca)
    Amyloidosis

4. Features associated with vasculitis

    Fever
    Digital arteritis (focal ischemic areas in nail fold, nail edge or digital pulp, gangrene, rare)
    Raynaud's phenomenon
    Skin lesions (rash and gangrene)
    Chronic leg ulcers
    Peripheral neuropathy (mononeuritis multiplex)
    Erosions in mucosa of gastrointestinal tract with hemorrhage
    Necrotizing arteritis involving mesenteric, coronary, renal vessels

5. RANGE OF MOTION: Indicate deficiencies in red on the following diagrams.

Figure 10-1.   (Cont'd)

NORMAL RANGE OF MOTION DIAGRAMS

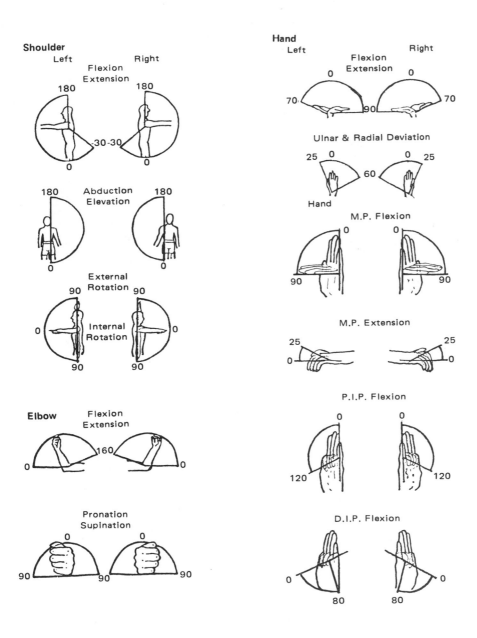

Figure 10–1.   (Cont'd)

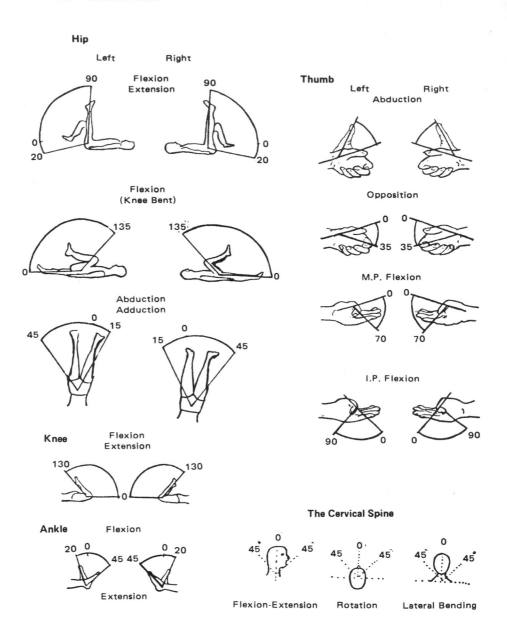

Figure 10-1.   (Cont'd)

patients, half of whom would have acupuncture and the other half some other type of treatment for the same disease.

CLINICAL RESULTS OF ACUPUNCTURE TREATMENTS FOR SPECIFIC CONDITIONS

Between April 1973 and April 1976, the Washington Acupuncture Center collected data on the results of acupuncture treatments on patients with 21 different medical disorders. Although the methods for collecting this information were not entirely objective and scientific, this is the largest study of acupuncture treatment results that has ever been made in the United States. The data are presented in the following table to give an indication of the effectiveness of acupuncture for treating the conditions listed.

RESULTS OF ACUPUNCTURE*

Condition Treated	Number of Cases	Number of Treatments	Improvement Significant	Slight	None
Alcoholism	205	6–20	174	10	21
Allergies	287	6–22	256	28	3
Arthritis					
Degenerative	2346	6–34	1955	367	24
Rheumatoid	827	10–66	634	177	16
Bursitis	683	6–16	584	81	18
Cerebral Palsy	42	10–55	30	10	2
Depression	872	6–28	686	183	3
Drug Addiction	68	6–37	52	2	14
Headaches	673	6–48	539	28	6
Insomnia	396	6–10	334	38	24
Lumbar Disc Syndrome	734	6–16	653	44	37
Menopausal Syndrome	266	6–24	251	12	3
Multiple Sclerosis	528	10–68	449	74	5
Neurosensory Deafness	569	10–60	293	204	72
Obesity	317	6–24	210	71	36
Pain, Chronic	2106	6–32	1847	227	32

RESULTS OF ACUPUNCTURE (Cont'd)

Condition Treated	Number of Cases	Number of Treatments	Improvement Significant	Slight	None
Paresis	475	10–182	293	102	80
Parkinsonism	123	10–34	58	38	27
Sexual Impotence	98	6–12	56	24	18
Tendonitis	207	6–24	130	46	31
Trigeminal Neuralgia	84	6–18	62	14	8
Whiplash Residuals	76	6–16	52	19	5

*These statistics were compiled by the Washington Acupuncture Center 4/73–4/76. Some patients were treated for more than one of these conditions.

FUTURE CLINICAL RESEARCH

Most clinical research in the United States is funded by drug companies, directly or indirectly through institutions supported by them. Since acupuncture is a substitute for drugs in treating many medical conditions, drug companies cannot be expected to fund acupuncture research. Acupuncture has become a political issue with various groups trying to discredit it for economic reasons.

As the government becomes increasingly concerned with reducing the cost and improving the quality of medical care in the United States, it should become more willing to fund research to compare acupuncture with more expensive and less effective treatments for chronic diseases which afflict millions of Americans. Insurance companies which pay for hospitalization may become interested in funding research on acupuncture analgesia for surgery to determine whether its use will reduce the time of post-operative hospitalization.

The acceptance of acupuncture by the medical community as a useful treatment modality depends on the publication of clinical research findings in medical journals and elsewhere. It is hoped that vested economic interests will not be able to prevent such research from being done or to suppress information about its results.

chapter 11

ACUPUNCTURIST AS A NEW HEALTH OCCUPATION*

SCOPE OF DUTIES

Job Description

An acupuncturist is a person with special medical training in the art of piercing the skin with fine needles at specific points to relieve pain, allergies, and depression, or improve function of various parts of the body.

Limitations of Function

An acupuncturist will only give acupuncture treatments to patients for whom acupuncture has been prescribed by a licensed physician who has examined the patient, diagnosed his ailments, determined that there is no better alternative treatment for him, and who supervises

---

*.With reference to American Medical Association Guidelines in 1974.

the acupuncturist closely enough to ascertain that aseptic technique is maintained.

Procedures for Assuring Medical Supervision

1. Each acupuncturist who is not a licensed physician should treat patients only under the supervision of a licensed physician who will be responsible for all aspects of the acupuncturist's treatment.

2. Acupuncturists should not be employed by non-physicians, unless the non-physician is a medical school, clinic, teaching hospital, or non-profit medical research institution.

3. An acupuncturist should not attempt to treat any ailment or give analgesia unless specifically asked to do so by the licensed physician who is supervising him.

4. Unless an acupuncturist speaks English fluently, he should only treat patients in the presence of an appropriate interpreter to facilitate his communication with his supervising physician and patients.

5. State Boards of Medical Examiners or other appropriate agencies should establish certification or registration procedures for acupuncturists, based on their having adequate verified training and passing both written and practical examinations.

6. Licensed physicians supervising acupuncturists should be on the premises and available to provide other medical treatment or consultation at all times during acupuncture treatment.

NEED

Since 1972 thousands of people have been treated by acupuncture in the United States for such conditions as arthritis, bursitis, headaches, neurogenic deafness, multiple sclerosis, cerebral palsy, allergies, addictions, depression, schizophrenia, and various pain syndromes for which no other treatment had been safe and effective. It has been used as the only analgesia for major surgery, tonsillectomies, and dental extractions.

Acupuncture Is Presently Being Performed by

1. Licensed physicians with adequate training and experience in acupuncture.

2.   Skilled but unlicensed and unregistered Oriental acupuncturists under the supervision of licensed physicians.

3.   Licensed physicians, many of Oriental ancestry, who have had very little training in acupuncture and do not yet have enough skill to treat neurogenic deafness and other neurologic disorders effectively.

4.   Skilled but unlicensed and unregistered Oriental acupuncturists practicing illegally without supervision and usually without aseptic techniques in Chinatowns of big cities and elsewhere.

5.   People with varying amounts of education who have had training and experience in acupuncture and who have been licensed as acupuncturists by such states as California, New York, and Nevada.

Why an Additional Type of Personnel Is Needed

Few licensed physicians in the United States have had much training in acupuncture. Although they can learn to give analgesia or treat some cases of arthritis after about 400 hours of training, it usually takes several years of experience to develop enough skill to treat neurologic disorders effectively. There is already such a shortage of physicians in the United States that we are importing large numbers of them from foreign countries. Even those from Oriental countries are unlikely to have had any training in acupuncture unless they have received their medical training in the People's Republic of China, where acupuncture has been taught to all medical students since 1955. It would take many years to develop enough licensed physicians to meet the patients' demands for acupuncture, even if more American medical schools start teaching acupuncture.

Few nurses, physician's assistants, or other paramedical personnel are able to perform acupuncture.

Patients Who Could Benefit from This Service

It is difficult to estimate the number of Americans now suffering from pain and disabilities which could be relieved safely and effectively by skilled acupuncture treatments. If the number of drugs sold for relief of pain, anxiety, depression, constipation, and nasal congestion each year is an indication, the majority of Americans could benefit from skilled acupuncture treatments during the next ten years.

In the People's Republic of China and in Taiwan, acupuncture is used as treatment for schizophrenia and other mental illnesses. Mental hospitals would probably employ large numbers of skilled acupuncturists if they were available.

Acupuncture can be especially useful in treating old and other chronically disabled people to enable them to become more self-sufficient. If Medicare were to pay for acupuncture treatments, the demand for them would be much greater than could possibly be met without a vigorous program to train non-physicians as well as physicians in acupuncture during the next ten years.

Impact on Existing Manpower Categories

Existing manpower categories cannot be assigned the functions of skilled acupuncturists because very few of them have any training in this medical technique.

The impact of creating this manpower category of "acupuncturist" on existing manpower categories might be as follows:

Licensed physicians.   Some physicians may choose to perform acupuncture themselves but more of them will prefer to employ skilled acupuncturists as technicians to relieve the pain and disabilities of their patients. Neurologists, psychiatrists, allergists, rheumatologists, orthopedists, surgeons, internists, otologists, and dentists would probably employ them.

Registered nurses and licensed practical nurses.   Some nurses might be trained in acupuncture for analgesia or relief of anxiety and depression.

Physiotherapists.   This group could receive training in acupuncture along with their regular training. Acupuncture can be considered a form of physiotherapy, but few if any physiotherapists in the United States are now trained in acupuncture.

Paramedics and ambulance personnel.   Such people could be trained to use acupuncture as a safe alternative to giving narcotics or other drugs for relief of pain after severe trauma.

Chiropractors.   Many chiropractors are already performing "acupressure" in an attempt to relieve pain by exerting pressure on acupuncture points. Some of them are already piercing the skin to perform acupuncture. Few of them have had more than a few weeks of training in acupuncture.

Views of Medical Specialists on the Potential Role of Acupuncture

Neurologists.   It is difficult for neurologists to believe that inserting fine needles superficially into the skin can have a therapeutic effect on nerve tissue. As they see the results of acupuncture on their patients with migraine headaches, trigeminal and other neuralgias, post-herpetic pain, multiple sclerosis, Parkinsonism, stroke residuals, cerebral palsy and other neurologic disorders, however, they become very much interested in acupuncture and want many of their patients to have it. Some of them are eager to master the technique themselves, but others would prefer to supervise technicians skilled in acupuncture.

Psychiatrists.   Since acupuncture is a safer treatment for mental illness than psychotropic drugs, electric shock, or psychosurgery, it is a good adjunct to psychotherapy. It has been found effective as treatment for anxiety, depression, schizophrenia, obesity, drug addiction, and alcoholism. Many psychiatrists have already attended seminars on acupuncture and seem optimistic about its use in treating their patients. One of the greatest demands for acupuncturists may come from mental health centers.

Orthopedists and Rheumatologists.   Many of them recognize acupuncture as a more conservative treatment than surgery for spinal disc syndromes and many other orthopedic problems. It is effective treatment for various types of arthritis for which drug therapy has been ineffective or damaging to the patient's general health. It can be given along with other forms of physiotherapy and may become an important therapeutic modality in orthopedic and rheumatology practice.

Surgeons.   Some have been impressed with films of the use of acupuncture as anesthesia for open heart surgery, brain surgery, and thyroidectomies in the People's Republic of China. It has already been used as analgesia for Caesarean section childbirth, tonsillectomies, thyroidectomies, and other surgery in the United States. Patients who are poor risks for chemical anesthesia can have surgery more safely with acupuncture analgesia if competent acupuncturists are available.

Anesthesiologists.   Many of them have shown great interest in acupuncture and some have learned to perform it themselves. It would be desirable and possible for all specialists in anesthesiology to learn acupuncture.

Obstetricians and Gynecologists.   Acupuncture is clearly the safest analgesia for childbirth and can also be used for many gynecological procedures. Acupuncturists could be very helpful to these medical specialists.

Otologists.   The greatest opposition to acupuncture has come from otologists. One famous otologist took brief training in acupuncture in China and then did some widely publicized acupuncture research in which he performed acupuncture on neurogenic deafness patients himself. (The only valid conclusion which can be drawn from his research is that he is not yet a skilled acupuncturist.)

Many otologists find it difficult to believe that acupuncture can improve hearing and are understandably concerned about the possibility of deaf people being exploited by quacks. Since otologists have no other safe and effective treatment to offer for neurogenic deafness, however, it seems important to do definitive research in which the acupuncture treatments are given by skilled acupuncturists who have had at least ten years of experience. People with neurogenic deafness get little help from hearing aids unless their word discrimination is improved by acupuncture.

Many patients with nerve deafness have already received effective acupuncture treatment by skilled acupuncturists under the supervision of licensed physicians. Treating nerve deafness, however, requires a much higher degree of acupuncture skill than giving analgesia. It is a technique that otologists should begin trying to master and should expect to take at least a year or two to become proficient in.

Allergists.   They tend to discount the effectiveness of acupuncture but are sometimes impressed with results and express interest in learning to perform it.

Other Physicians.   Every physician is frequently confronted with problems of pain, anxiety, and depression that might be effectively and safely relieved by acupuncture. There is considerable evidence that acupuncture could substantially reduce the consumption of narcotics and other dangerous drugs now used to relieve these problems.

Public Acceptance of Acupuncturists

Since the first acupuncture clinic was established in the United States in 1972, patients have been seeking acupuncture treatments for chronic diseases for which there is no safe and effective alternative treatment. Many of them have experienced relief from pain and disabilities they had been told they would have to tolerate for the rest of their lives. Their physicians and friends have seen the results of acupuncture. Unless the American Medical Association supports making skilled acupuncture treatments under the supervision of licensed physicians available to the general public, too many patients will seek acupuncture from unsupervised and unlicensed practitioners of this Oriental art.

EDUCATION AND TRAINING

Acupuncture should be included in the curricula of all medical schools because it is useful in all medical specialties except pathology and radiology. Every physician could benefit from knowing how to relieve pain, anxiety, and depression without drugs. Dentists, dental hygienists, nurses, physiotherapists, paramedics, and other health professionals could be taught acupuncture during their regular course of study. The prerequisite courses for acupuncture training should include anatomy and physiology.

Acupuncture is also an excellent subject for Continuing Medical Education courses for physicians and paramedical personnel.

Educational Setting

The educational setting for training in acupuncture is not dependent on the availability of heavy, expensive, or elaborate equipment. It should, therefore, be possible to teach acupuncture in any classroom where there is a padded table for patients, chairs for self-practice, wall charts of acupuncture points, an acupuncture manikin, small point-finding instruments, and a supply of properly sterilized acupuncture needles. Clinical experience could be in any type of hospital or physician's office.

Tuition

Because of the great demand for skilled acupuncture treatments, an acupuncturist can expect to earn a good salary. Many people have written to the Acupuncture Institute requesting a course in acupuncture. As government officials become aware of its potential for reducing the disabilities of the aged and other people, government funding of acupuncture training is a possibility. The Department of Health, Education and Welfare paid the tuition for one of its psychiatrists to take a 400-hour course at the Acupuncture Institute in Washington, D.C.

Interest of Young People

Many young people who have a negative attitude about the delivery of health care and the training of health professionals in the United States seem greatly interested in acupuncture. I receive many invitations to speak to classes of high school students and am impressed with their eagerness to learn as much about it as possible.

EMPLOYMENT AND CAREER OPPORTUNITIES

Salaries I now pay the skilled Oriental acupuncturists who work under my supervision are higher than what state and federal government agencies pay licensed physicians. As the supply of acupuncturists increases, their salaries may decrease, but it seems likely that, for many years to come, the demand for their services at a high rate of compensation will continue.

Settings for Employment

Acupuncturists may be employed in General Hospitals to provide:

1. Analgesia for surgery and other painful procedures.
2. Analgesia for post-operative pain.
3. Analgesia for accident victims.
4. Analgesia for patients with chronic pain syndromes, such as cancer, arthritis, and trigeminal neuralgia.
5. Relief from allergic symptoms.
6. Relief from depression and anxiety.

Mental hospitals, mental health clinics, and physicians' offices may also employ acupuncturists.

Professional Certification

Several states, including California, New York, and Nevada, have already established a procedure for evaluating the credentials of acupuncturists and giving them written and practical examinations. As courses for training acupuncturists are established, appropriate procedures can be set up for certifying American-trained acupuncturists.

Mobility

Upward mobility within the discipline should depend on the skill attained with experience and continuing education. Mobility from one medical specialty to another should be facilitated by the acupuncturist's taking courses related to the medical specialty in which he wants to use his skill.

There is no reason that the certification of acupuncturists should not be essentially the same in every state with reciprocity between the states.

ACUPUNCTURE TREATMENT OF SPECIFIC CONDITIONS

chapter 12

GENERAL PRINCIPLES
OF TREATMENT

Anyone who has read the previous chapters of this book knows that acupuncture is not a "cure-all," has many limitations, and should not be used to mask symptoms of undiagnosed diseases or to delay necessary surgery, chemotherapy, antibiotics, or other effective medications. It is mostly for analgesia and treatment of chronic, thoroughly diagnosed disorders.

CLASSIFICATION OF MEDICAL PROBLEMS

Part 2 may be used as a reference book for determining which points to use in clinical practice. To make it as useful as possible to people with varying educational backgrounds, the medical problems for which acupuncture might be considered are listed alphabetically in the index in popular language as well as being classified by body systems and listed in medical terminology in the following chapters.

Many diseases involve more than one body system and may be classified under several different medical specialties. Almost every disease, for instance, involves pain, depression, fatigue, and insomnia. It would be repetitious to include treatment of these common symptoms under each of the body system categories. In a sense, all pain is psychological or at least neurologic. If we did not have nerves and brains, we could not perceive pain from an arthritic joint or an inflamed muscle. When one has a painful disease, it is natural to be depressed about the persistence of pain and the restriction of activities. There is also the fear that the pain may last the rest of one's life or even become worse. Depression may follow discovery that one has a progressive disease with little likelihood of cure or remission, even if it is not painful. If pain is episodic, as in trigeminal neuralgia or migraine headaches, a person is likely to have considerable anxiety about when the next episode will occur. Insomnia usually follows pain, depression and anxiety. Obesity, alcoholism, drug addiction, or anorexia may represent different people's attempts to deal with similar problems of depression, anxiety, and frustration. Almost every disease syndrome has psychological components, and it is usually impossible to determine whether psychological problems caused the disease or the disease caused the psychological problems.

Allergies are involved in symptoms of every body system and are usually closely associated with emotional problems. Some physicians have found reasons to think that such apparently different conditions as arthritis and hyperactivity may both be dependent on food allergies.

No classification of medical disorders seems satisfactory. Each body system or organ is dependent on the others. Many people who read this book will object to the listing of some specific disorder under a specific body system and think it should have been placed in a different category. Acupuncturists have suggested that this problem could be avoided simply by discussing each condition in alphabetical order without regard to body systems. My American medical colleagues, however, have urged me to classify disorders by body systems in spite of overlapping problems.

As explained in Chapter 6, the most competent acupuncturists refuse to limit their practice to one special part of the body. Acupuncturists who specialize in treating only a specific organ or giving analgesia for a restricted area are regarded as acupuncture technicians. Even acupuncture technicians, however, should be concerned with the patient's general health and the effect that each treatment seems to have on it, as well as on the specific part of the body being treated.

The items in parentheses after items listed in the index should not be considered synonymous with these conditions. Parenthetical items should be referred to for information about treatment of listed conditions.

USE OF ACUPUNCTURE PRESCRIPTIONS

The acupuncture points for treating specific conditions listed here include those given in Chinese textbooks[1-9] and those used by acupuncturists at the Washington Acupuncture Center. These specific points should be used as guidelines in selecting the points for each treatment rather than as formulas to be followed precisely. They may be used bilaterally or unilaterally. Not all of them need to be used for each treatment or for each patient. They can be supplemented with other points to be determined by the acupuncturist on the basis of his evaluation of the patient and past experience.

Patients can be treated with acupuncture for several different ailments at the same time. Some points, such as Colon 4 and Stomach 36, are included in the lists of standard points for treating many different disorders. In determining how to treat a multiple-problem patient, however, great skill is required. Such patients may not be able to tolerate more than ten needles per treatment. The points for these should be chosen very carefully.

One of a patient's disorders may show improvement long before another does. Insomnia or nasal congestion, for instance, may be relieved after the first treatment, but the patient's stroke residuals may require twenty or more treatments for maximal improvement. Even though a symptom is relieved after the first treatment, at least two needles should be inserted for this symptom on the two following treatments to prevent its recurrence.

If a patient has sensory loss in an extremity, the first sensation to return during acupuncture is likely to be pain. Although this is an encouraging sign, a patient may need considerable reassurance, and perhaps even a few needles, to cope with it.

Some of the acupuncture points listed for relieving certain types of pain can be used effectively as pressure points for temporary relief of pain. A thin, blunt instrument, or even a finger, may be used for this purpose. Probes, electrode pads of TES (transcutaneous electric stimulation) or point-finding instruments may be similarly used. This is a safe procedure but does not usually produce lasting relief of pain or other symptoms. Chapters 2 and 3 should be referred to for point location.

Although there is general uniformity in the location of acupuncture points on all human bodies, there is great variation in the size and shape of different people. The system of measuring body inches is probably used unconsciously by surgeons and other physicians, but it may not seem adequate to the beginning acupuncturist. Electric point-finding instruments may be helpful and are now available in the United States.

The techniques and precautions described in Part I, Chapter 8, as well as the information given in other chapters, should be well understood before attempting to give acupuncture treatment.

ADVICE FOR PATIENTS

Oriental acupuncturists believe that patients will derive more benefit from acupuncture if they avoid cold temperatures, iced drinks, spicy food, alcohol, and coffee at least until their series of treatments has been completed. Nutritional advice should be given to all acupuncture patients, and they should be urged to continue nutritional therapy after completing their acupuncture treatments.

GENERAL REFERENCES FOR CHAPTERS   12–21

1. Silverstein, Martin E.; Chang, I-Lok; and Mason, Nathaniel. (translators), *Acupuncture and Moxibustion, A Handbook for the Barefoot Doctors of China*. New York: Schocken Books, 1975.

2. Academy of Traditional Chinese Medicine. *An Outline of Chinese Acupuncture*. Peking: Foreign Language Press, 1975.

3. Anonymous. *An Explanatory Book of the Newest Illustrations of Acupuncture Points*. Hong Kong: Medicine and Health Publishing Co., 1974.

4. Cheong, W.C.; and Yang, C.P. *Synopsis of Chinese Acupuncture*. Hong Kong: The Light Publishing Co., 1974.

5. Anonymous. *An Outline of Chinese Acupuncture* (In Chinese). Peking: People's Hygiene Press, 1972.

6. Kao, Wu. *Finest Writings on Acupuncture* (In Chinese). Shanghi: Technical Scientific Publishing Company, 1978.

7. Traditional Chinese Medical Institute. *A Concise Acupuncture Textbook* (In Chinese). Peking: People's Medical Publisher, 1978.

8. Chang, Kui-Sun. *Anthology on Acupuncture* (In Chinese). Lanchow City, China: Gansu People's Publishing Co., 1978.

9. Shanghi College of Traditional Chinese Medicine. *Acupuncture and Moxibustion Textbook* (In Chinese). Peking: People's Health Publishing Company, 1974.

chapter 13

ANESTHESIA
OR ANALGESIA

The English words *anesthesia* and *analgesia* are misleading to describe the freedom from surgical or obstetrical pain which can be produced by acupuncture. If *analgesia* is defined as "insensibility to pain without loss of consciousness," it is a more appropriate word than *anesthesia*, which is defined as "insensibility, general or local, induced by anesthetic agents; and loss of sensation of neurogenic or psychogenic origin." Acupuncture analgesia is the term, therefore, which will be found in this book most frequently.

Acupuncture does not alter the level of consciousness or produce numbness of any part of the body. The patient under acupuncture analgesia remains able to converse and cooperate with the surgical or obstetrical team. Obstetrical patients are aware of uterine contractions and able to use their muscles to expel the fetus. Surgical patients can tell when incisions are made but do not perceive them as painful. There is no loss of memory, as in hypnosis or general anesthesia, and no paresthesia comparable to the sensations following local anesthesia.[1]

ADVANTAGES

Most operating room deaths and cardiac arrests in the United States are caused by chemical anesthesia rather than by surgery.[2] Surgeons and anesthesiologists should all be eager to have a safer alternative available. Patients who are poor anesthetic risks because of heart, liver, or kidney disease, tolerate acupuncture analgesia well. Infants and elderly people are also good candidates for acupuncture analgesia.

Although acupuncture does not alter the level of consciousness, it can be used to induce a feeling of well-being or calmness to allay the fear and apprehensiveness most patients feel before surgery. It also seems to reduce the bleeding during surgical procedures and the incidence of shock. Post-operative patients are spared from nausea and the difficulties with urinating and defecating which frequently follow chemical anesthesia. Acupuncture analgesia does not mask symptoms as chemical anesthetics and analgesics do. The patient remains aware of his symptoms but acupuncture diminishes them to a tolerable level.

Post-operative pain does not usually occur for several hours after acupuncture analgesia has been terminated. Then acupuncture can be used again instead of narcotics and seldom needs to be repeated more than once or twice. Some acupuncturists leave small needles superficially inserted for several days to give post-operative pain relief. Others give regular daily acupuncture treatments, leaving the needles in place for 20 minutes as many days as necessary.

DISADVANTAGES

The main disadvantage of acupuncture analgesia is that it is less reliable than chemical analgesia or anesthesia. In some cases, acupuncture analgesia cannot be induced or becomes inadequate during a surgical procedure. It may not produce the relaxation desirable for some abdominal surgery. For this reason, backup chemical anesthetics and analgesics should be available whenever possible.[3]

The success of acupuncture analgesia depends on the skill of the acupuncturist. Although there are few skilled acupuncturists in the United States at present, it takes less time to train a physician, nurse, or medical technician to perform acupuncture analgesia than to teach him how to give acupuncture treatments for chronic diseases or to give chemical anesthesia or analgesia.

If training in acupuncture analgesia were made a Continuing Medical Education requirement for all anesthesiologists, acupuncture analgesia would soon be available in all American hospitals. This technique could even be taught in nursing schools and medical schools. "Acupuncture analgesia technicians" could be a category of paramedical personnel with less educational requirements.

One of the disadvantages of acupuncture analgesia is that more time is required to prepare a patient for it than to prepare him for chemical analgesia or anesthesia. If acupuncture is to be used for elective surgery, the acupuncturist should become acquainted with the patient ahead of time, answer his questions, explain the surgical as well as acupuncture procedures, allay his fears, and experiment with needles or acupressure to determine the points which are most effective for producing analgesia in the desired area. Unless the acupuncturist can produce analgesia for a patient by this experimental procedure the day before the surgery, he should not attempt to use acupuncture for this patient's surgery.[4] He should try to obtain the services of a more skillful acupuncturist, if possible, or notify the surgeon that he will have to rely on chemical anesthesia.

If a patient is unduly apprehensive and does not respond to verbal assurances or acupuncture for relief of his anxiety and fear, a mild sedative or narcotic may be used as a pre-operative medication along with acupuncture. No one, except an infant too young to give verbal consent, should be forced to have acupuncture analgesia. Obtaining the cooperation of the patient is very important, although acupuncture has been used successfully for surgery on babies and animals.

If a patient complains of pain after a surgical procedure is in process, local anesthesia can be given as indicated. If the patient becomes so uncomfortable that he asks to be put to sleep, this can be done with chemical anesthesia at any time. Acupuncture does not interfere with the effectiveness of general or local anesthesia.

The actual induction of acupuncture analgesia takes about 20 minutes, not much longer than chemical anesthesia induction. In most cases, electro-acupuncture instruments must remain attached to all acupuncture needles during the entire procedure, but these can usually be kept away from the surgical field. The more skilled the acupuncturist, the fewer the needles required. In China, major surgical procedures have been performed with only one acupuncture needle as analgesia without electric potentiation. The beginning acupuncturist, however, may need to insert more than 10 needles to obtain adequate analgesia for surgery. Using acupuncture points on the ears, feet, and hands keeps the needles and electro-acupuncture instruments from interfering with the surgical field.

MECHANISM OF ACUPUNCTURE ANALGESIA

As was explained in Chapter 5, acupuncture at various points on the body can stimulate the brain, pituitary gland, and other structures to produce endorphins, morphine-like biochemicals. Their analgesic properties are similar to those of morphine and other narcotics but they do not cause addiction and are non-toxic.

Several studies have been performed to compare acupuncture analgesia with hypnotic states in which a person is able to tolerate surgery without chemical anesthesia.[5,6] Hypnosis and acupuncture have similar advantages over chemical analgesics and anesthetics, but hypnosis is much less reliable than acupuncture and cannot be used for infants. Even the most competent hypnotists are usually unable to induce deep enough hypnosis for surgery unless they have hypnotized the patient many times before. It is also difficult for a hypnotist to keep a patient under deep hypnosis long enough for the surgery to be completed. Acupuncturists do not attempt to use hypnotic techniques. Oriental acupuncturists unable to speak English are able to give English-speaking people acupuncture analgesia. Interpreters serving such acupuncturists need no training or skill in hypnosis.

TECHNIQUES AND EQUIPMENT

The same type of thin (usually 30 gauge) stainless steel solid needles that are used for acupuncture treatments are used for acupuncture analgesia. In general, the points which are used to relieve chronic pain in a specific area are the points of choice for analgesia, except that points near the surgical field should be avoided. To obtain enough analgesia for surgery, it is usually necessary to potentiate the effect of the acupuncture needles by twirling them continually or by attaching electronic instruments to them to deliver a current of about 200 microamperes, with a pulsating wave at 200 per minute frequency during the entire procedure. As more Americans become proficient in acupuncture, however, it can be expected that fewer of them will require electro-acupuncture instruments for potentiation, especially for surgery requiring less than half an hour for completion. Potentiation techniques can be added at any time during the procedure and will usually increase the depth of analgesia or prolong an analgesic effect which is beginning to wear off. Sometimes it is effective to insert more acupuncture needles during a surgical procedure if the analgesia becomes inadequate or if the patient becomes apprehensive or uncomfortable.

Besides the acupuncture points for analgesia of specific areas of the body, it is often desirable to use points for relieving anxiety and promoting a feeling of well-being. These should usually be inserted for 20 minutes the evening before surgery as well as for at least 20 minutes before the actual surgery begins. If they are inserted during surgery, it will probably take 20 minutes for them to be effective. This much delay in the midst of a surgical procedure is generally undesirable.

Injecting 0.5 cc. of 2% procaine, or a similar local anesthetic, at appropriate acupuncture points is a technique that has been found successful in some cases.[7] Acupuncture points for such injections need not be near the surgical field. Needles used for this purpose can be left in place and electrodes attached to them for electric potentiation during surgery. Injections of morphine, Demerol, or other narcotics in varying doses have been used in a similar manner. Such drug potentiation, however, is usually unnecessary if the acupuncturist is highly skilled. There have even been some reports that injecting local anesthetics and narcotics at acupuncture points is less effective than inserting regular acupuncture needles without any type of potentiation.

Since acupuncture does not give the level of muscle relaxation which can be attained by chemical anesthesia, it should not be depended on for abdominal surgery requiring extensive visceral manipulation even though it has been used successfully for appendectomies and Caesarian section deliveries.[8]

The theoretical principles of vital energy transmission are used in determining which acupuncture points might be effective for the anticipated surgery. Acupuncture points on meridians passing directly through, or in the vicinity of, the surgical area are usually selected. An attempt is made to use points on these meridians which are as far away from the surgical field as possible.

SPECIFIC POINTS FOR SPECIFIC PROCEDURES[9]

For facial, dental, and pharyngeal surgery, points on Meridian Co (colon) are used because it is thought to pass through the major supraclavicular fossa to the neck, chin, teeth, and lips to the nostrils. The *Yang* meridians (Co, St, SI, UB, Me, and GB) and Meridian Li all pass through the head area. Points on these meridians in lower parts of the body are therefore used for anesthesia of head areas. Most meridian lines are regarded as passing from distal parts of the body toward more proximal areas and from superficial to deep locations. For this reason the origin (*Yuan*) and accumulating (*Lo*) loci are often used. For example, Co 4 and Li 3, the origin *loci* of their respective meridians, are often included for visceral as well as head and neck surgery.

Hsia Ho loci are points where the *Yang* meridians of the legs are thought to accumulate energy. Their points on the legs are often used for anesthetizing areas near the viscera they are thought to influence. Points frequently used for this purpose are St 36 and 38, UB 54, and GB 34.

Chiao Ho loci are points where two or more meridians are thought to meet. There are more than 100 of these located in different parts of the body. For example, SI 18 is the meeting point of Meridians SI (small intestine) and ME (metabolism). Sp 6 is the meeting place of the spleen and kidney meridians.

Acupuncture point Va 4 of the vascular meridian has been found useful for calming patients who become apprehensive during surgical procedures. It is supposed to relieve any heart palpitation or dyspnea which might develop.

For thyroidectomy, the superficial nerves are stimulated through Co 18. Branches from the trigeminal nerve are stimulated through SI 18 for head surgery anesthesia.

Precise localization of the acupuncture points is essential. From the experience and records of clinical practice, there are still some individual differences in the localization of acupuncture points, especially in people who have had previous surgery or who have deformities. Electronic equipment for localizing acupuncture points is helpful for determining exact locations for acupuncture anesthesia.

Auricular acupuncture points corresponding to different regions of the body are outlined in the chapter on "Special Acupuncture Points." In performing an appendectomy, for instance, the representative acupuncture points on the ear for the appendix and abdominal area are used. In performing a thyroidectomy, the representative acupuncture points for the areas of the throat and neck are used. In arm surgery, the representative point for the elbow area is used. In surgery involving the removal of a gastric or duodenal ulcer, the representative points for the digestive organs are used.

For ear needle anesthesia, the specific acupuncture point corresponding to the surgical area is supplemented with coordinating acupuncture points based on meridian theory. For example, Meridian Lu (lung) is considered to dominate all the skin structure of the body. For skin surgery, therefore, the acupuncture points of Meridian Lu are used to coordinate with the specific ear point to induce the anesthetic effect. The kidney is considered to dominate all the bones of the body.

For bone surgery, the acupuncture points of Meridian Ki are used. For reducing muscle tension, the coordinating points of Meridian Sp are chosen because the spleen is thought to dominate the muscles.

Some of the most frequently used meridian acupuncture points for anesthesia of specific areas are as follows:

Eyes:	Co 4 · St 2
Ears:	Co 4 · Me 3 and 17
Nose:	Co 4 and 20 · St 2
Upper Teeth:	Co 4 · St 6, 7 and 44
Lower Teeth:	Co 4 · St 5 and 6
Throat:	Co 4 · St 6 and 44
Esophagus:	Co 4 · Va 6
Urethra:	St 36 · Sp 6 · Sx 4 · Br 2
Uterus:	St 36 · Sp 6 · Li 3 · Br 4

In 1975, a group of Peking physicians reported the following combinations of acupuncture points which they felt could be used successfully for specific operations.[10]

Intracranial surgery

Meridian points:	Co 4 · Va 6 · SI 18 · St 43 · Li 3 · UB 2 · GB 2, 8, and 41 · Br 20 · Me 21
Auricular points:	Shenmen · Kidney · Forehead · Sympathy · Lung

Eye surgery

Meridian points:	Co 4 · Me 5 · Va 6 · UB 2 · SI 6 · GB 14 and 37 · Li 3 · St 1, 2, and 7
Auricular points:	Shenmen · Lung · Eye · Eye I · Eye II · Liver · Kidney · Sympathy · Forehead

Normal childbirth

Meridian points:	Co 4 · Va 6 · Sp 6 and 9 · Li 3 and 6 · St 36 and 44
Auricular points:	Genitalia · Urethra · Hip · Abdomen · Lumbar · Uterus · Sympathy

Surgery on the ear

    Meridian points: Co 4 · Va 6 · St 2, 3, and 44

Nose surgery

    Meridian points: Co 4 and 20 · St 2 and 3 · Va 6 · SI 3

    Auricular points: Forehead · Internal Nose · External Nose · Shenmen · Sympathy · Lung

Maxillary surgery

    Meridian points: St 2 and 3 · Co 4, 11, and 20 · Me 5 and 6 · Va 6 · St 36

    Auricular points: Maxilla · Forehead · External Nose · Internal Nose · Shenmen · Sympathy · Kidney

Laryngeal surgery

    Meridian points: Co 4 · Me 6

    Auricular points: Pharynx · Larynx · Neck · Lung · Kidney · Shenmen · Sympathy

Tonsillectomies

    Meridian points: Co 4 · Me 6 · Li 3 · Ki 7 · Va 6

    Auricular points: Pharynx · Larynx · Tonsil

Mandibular area surgery

    Meridian points: Co 4 · St 40 and 43 · GB 38 and 43 · UB 60 · Li 3 · Sp 4 · Va 6

Cleft palate surgery

    Meridian points: Co 4 and 20 · Va 4 and 6 · GB 38 · St 6, 7 and 40 · Br 26 · Sx 24 · SI 18

Neck surgery [including thyroid]

    Meridian points: Co 4 and 18 · Va 6 · St 6 · GB 31

    Auricular points: Shenmen · Sympathy · Lung · Neck · Pharynx · Larynx

Chest surgery

    Meridian points: Co 4 and 14 · Va 4 and 6 · Me 5, 6, 8, and 14 · Br 11 and 13

    Auricular points: Shenmen · Sympathy · Lung · Kidney · Thoracic · Heart · Esophagus

Stomach and intestines

    Meridian points: St 36 and 37 · Me 17 · Va 6

    Auricular points: Abdomen · Shenmen · Sympathy · Colon · Stomach · Lung · Diaphragm · Small Intestine

Gallbladder and biliary duct surgery

    Meridian points: St 36 · Sp 6

    Auricular points: Gall Bladder · Liver · Stomach · Diaphragm · Lung · Sympathy · Shenmen · Pancreas · Abdomen

Splenectomy

    Meridian points: St 36 · Sp 4 and 6 · Li 3 and 13 · Sx 15 · Va 4 · Co 4

    Auricular points: Spleen · Lung · Sympathy · Shenmen · Abdomen

Appendectomy

    Meridian points: St 36 · GB 20

    Auricular points: Appendix · Abdomen · Lung · Colon · Small Intestine · Sympathy · Shenmen

Herniorrhaphy

    Meridian points: St 36 · GB 28 · UB 18 and 25 · Sp 15

    Auricular points: Abdomen · Sympathy · Knee

Gynecological and obstetrical surgery

    Meridian points: St 36 · Li 6 · GB 26 and 34 · Sp 6 and 9 · Br 2 and 4 · UB 32 and 33

    Auricular points: Shenmen · Sympathy · Uterus · Gonads · Lung · Abdomen · Kidney

Urological surgery

    Meridian points: GB 27, 28, and 38 · UB 34 and 60 · Ki 3 · St 43 · Li 3 and 5 · Sp 3 and 6 · Co 4 · Me 5 · SI 3 · Va 4 · Sx 3 and 4

    Auricular points: Shenmen · Sympathy · Lung · Kidney · Urinary Bladder · Abdomen

Hemorrhoidectomy

> Meridian points: UB 30 and 49
>
> Auricular points: Rectum • Lung • Sympathy • Shenmen

Shoulder and elbow surgery or manipulation

> Meridian points: Va 4 and 6 • Co 4, 15, and 18 • Lu 6 • Me 5
>
> Auricular points: Shenmen • Sympathy • Shoulder • Lung • Kidney • Elbow

Arm and hand surgery

> Meridian points: Co 4, 11, and 15 • He 2 and 3 • Lu 2, 5, and 10 • Me 9, 5, and 13 • GB 34 • UB 54 • St 36
>
> Auricular points: Shenmen • Sympathy • Shoulder • Lung • Kidney • Elbow

Hip and lower extremity surgery

> Meridian points: St 31, 36, 40, and 44 • UB 40, 59, and 60 • GB 30, 31, 34, 39, and 43 • Li 3 and 5 • Sp 6, 9, 10, and 12 • Ki 3
>
> Auricular points: Shenmen • Sympathy • Lung • Knee • Hip • Buttocks • Kidney • Toes • Ankle

Lumbar laminectomy

> Meridian points: Co 4 • Me 5 • Va 6 • Br 3 and 4
>
> Auricular points: Shenmen • Sympathy • Lung • Kidney • Lumbar spine

For anesthesia as for acupuncture treatment, the acupuncture points apparently remain effective even if the organ after which their meridian is named has been removed.

Besides the points for analgesia listed in this chapter, the points on the soles of the feet, the face, and some of the extraordinary points may be useful for analgesia in some cases. Diagrams for locating these points are included in Chapter 3.

REFERENCES FOR CHAPTER   13

1.   Wen, W. "Acupuncture Anesthesia in China." *Comparative Medicine East and West* (5) (Summer 1977): 185–8.

2. Gordon, T.; Larson, C.P. Jr.; and Prestivich, R. "Unexpected Cardiac Arrest during Anesthesia and Surgery." *Journal of the American Medical Association* 236 (1976): 2758–2760.

3. Murphy, T.M.; and Bonica, J.J. "Acupuncture Analgesia and Anesthesia." *Archives of Surgery* 112(7) (July 1977): 896–902.

4. Diamond, E.G. "Acupuncture Anesthesia: Western Medicine and Chinese Traditional Medicine." *Journal of the American Medical Association* 218 (1971): 1558–1563.

5. Frost, E.A. "Acupuncture and Hypnosis. Apples and Oranges." *New York State Journal of Medicine* 78 (11) (September 1978): 1768–1772.

6. Mac Hovec, F.J.; and Man, C.S. "Acupuncture and Hypnosis Compared: Fifty–eight Cases." *American Journal of Clinical Hypnosis* 21 (1) (July 1978): 45–47.

7. Bull, G.M. "Acupuncture Anesthesia." *Lancet* 2 (1973): 417–418.

8. Anonymous. *Acupuncture Anesthesia*, 15–65, Roerig Division of Pfeizer Pharmaceuticals, 1974.

9. Anonymous. *The Principles and Practical Use of Acupuncture Anesthesia*, 168–307. Hong Kong: Medicine and Health Publishing Co., 1974.

10. Academy of Traditional Chinese Medicine. *An Outline of Chinese Acupuncture*, pp. 290–298. Peking: Foreign Language Press, 1975.

chapter 14

ALLERGIES

Allergies are excessively adverse reactions to certain substances a person is exposed to by skin contact, inhalation, ingestion, or injection. Hay fever, bronchial asthma, angioneurotic edema, anaphylactic shock, many skin rashes, and some cases of nausea and vomiting are allergic reactions. Even some cases of arthritis, colitis, and hyperactivity are thought to have an allergic component.

The substance to which the person is allergic is called the *antigen*, and the blood components produced in response to antigens are called *antibodies*. Much research is being done on antigen-antibody reactions in relation to the body's immune mechanisms. The Washington Acupuncture Center has engaged in such research with the Microbiology Department of George Washington University Medical School to evaluate the regulatory effect of acupuncture on this body process.

Most people with allergy problems are allergic to so many different substances that it is impossible to avoid contact with all of them. Such common allergens as dust and pollen cannot be completely avoided, but allergic reactions to these are usually much less severe than allergic reactions to drugs. Any drug is a potential allergen which may produce a life-threatening allergic reaction. Even antihistamines produce severe allergic reactions for some people. For this reason, it is important for people with allergies to take as few drugs as possible and to keep an accurate account of past allergic reactions to drugs.

Nobody is allergic to acupuncture because no chemical is injected into the body. Acupuncture can reduce a person's allergic responses to most common allergens enough to relieve and prevent hay fever, asthma, some cases of dermatitis, indigestion, and diarrhea. It can also be used as an alternative to potentially allergenic drugs for relieving pain and treating many diseases. Acupuncture, however, should not be depended on as the only treatment for severe allergic reactions to drugs and anaphylactic shock. A person should not take a drug he knows he's allergic to expecting that acupuncture will prevent allergic reaction.

People with allergic tendencies should avoid contact with known allergens as much as possible and supplement their diets with large amounts of Vitamins A, C, and Pantothenate. As mentioned in Chapter 7, nobody is allergic to vitamins, but some people are allergic to the fillers used to make vitamin tablets and capsules. Changing the brand of vitamins can usually relieve this problem.

Although allergies may be classified as respiratory, food, drug, or dermatologic, people with severe allergic diatheses may show allergic symptoms in many different parts of the body. Instead of treating specific allergic symptoms, acupuncture can be used to reduce a person's general tendency to react allergically.

The treatments of specific allergic symptoms, such as asthma, chronic siunusitis, colitis, and contact dermatitis are discussed under those headings. The points to use for reducing a person's general tendency to react allergically are as follows:

Meridian points: Br 10 and 14 · UB 10, 11, 13, 14, 25, 26, 38, 54, and 57 · Sx 6, 12, 14, 17, and 22 · Lu 1 and 7 · St 25, 36, 40 · Co 4 and 11 · GB 20 and 30 · SI 14 · Li 10 · Va 6 · Me 5 · Ki 3 · Sp 6

Auricular points: Lung · Internal Nose · Maxillary Sinus · Stomach · Small Intestine · Liver

Not all of these points should be used for each treatment. The points selected should be bilateral in most cases, and the needles left in them for about 20 minutes. Electric and infrared potentiation may be beneficial.

Although nasal congestion is usually relieved during the first treatment, other symptoms may require more treatments, usually at least six for lasting relief. Some patients may need to have another series of four to six treatments each year at the beginning of their allergy seasons.

A person who has been taking desensitizing injections can usually discontinue them after a course of acupuncture treatments. Many people have had severe adverse reactions to some of their desensitizing injections because of contamination or overdose and have found such injections inadequate for preventing their allergic reactions.

If a patient has been taking cortisone or its derivatives over a long period of time as treatment for allergy, however, he should be advised to reduce this medication very slowly no matter how effective the acupuncture treatments are. The physiological dependence on such drugs is so serious that a life-threatening adrenal crisis could result from abrupt withdrawal. Vitamin C (3 gm.) and Pantothenate (300 mg.) daily should be prescribed to help restore function of the patient's adrenal glands after suppression by corticoid therapy.

ASTHMA

Asthma is a disease process involving widespread narrowing of the bronchi and is associated with wheezing and often dyspnea at rest. The bronchial narrowing is a response to inhaled, ingested, or parenterally administered antigens. Asthma may also be induced by bacterial or viral infections and is apparently a manifestation of an allergic response to some allergen produced by the infecting organism.

Although asthma may be a life threatening disease, many physicians consider emotional factors significant in precipitating acute exacerbations. We might say that they cause an imbalance of *Yin-Yang* energy in the respiratory system making the patient more sensitive to allergens.

Evaluation of asthma patients prior to acupuncture treatment should exclude an infective or parenteral basis for the disease. A chest X-ray will help to exclude causes of wheezing, such as airway obstruction by a foreign body or neoplasm. Consideration should also be given to more rare causes of wheezing, such as serotonin-producing tumors. Most patients seeking acupuncture treatment for asthma, however, have had the disease for several years and adequate diagnostic studies to rule out etiology requiring surgical or antibiotic treatment.

The first acupuncture treatment will often relieve an acute exacerbation, but a course of six to ten treatments should be given for lasting relief. It is not necessary that the patient have asthma symptoms at the time he takes acupuncture treatments for it.

If a person has been taking cortisone or one of its derivatives for a long time, the drug may have suppressed his adrenal glands to the point that he will develop an adrenal crisis if he stops taking the drug abruptly. These drugs should only be discontinued gradually over a period of months under the supervision of a physician, even if the asthma has been completely relieved by acupuncture. Unfortunately, too few physicians who prescribe cortisone and its derivatives explain that these drugs may create a dependence more serious than heroin-dependence.

The classical acupuncture points used for treating asthma include the following:

For an acute attack

Meridian points: St 3, 4, 5, 6, and 40 · Me 3, 4, 5, and 6 · UB 12 and 13 · Lu 5 · Sx 17

Auricular points: Lung · Shenmen · Sympathy

For chronic asthma

Meridian points: UB 12, 23, and 38 · Sx 6, 12, 14, and 22 · Lu 7 · Br 14 · Co 4 · GB 20 · SI 14

Auricular points: Lung · Internal Nose · Maxillary Sinus

HAY FEVER

Hay fever is an allergic reaction to inhaled pollens and is characterized by sneezing, itching, and watery discharge from the nose and eyes. It is most prevalent in early spring when tree pollen is spread, early summer when grass pollen is spread, and in early fall when weed pollen is spread. In the fall, molds and decaying vegetation produce allergenic spores. Animal dander, dust, broken insect parts, and various chemical air pollutants can cause allergic reactions like hay fever any time of the year.

It is possible to test for specific allergies with skin tests and then give injections in an attempt to decrease sensitivity. Such treatment, however, is prolonged, painful, sometimes dangerous, and often ineffective. The desensitizing liquids may contain contaminants or too much of the allergen to be well tolerated by the patient.

Exposure to allergens can be reduced by avoiding contact with animals, house plants, and feather pillows, by staying inside with air conditioning during allergy seasons, and by removing dust-collecting household items, such as rugs and draperies.

Emotional problems aggravate hay fever and other allergic reactions. When a person feels happy and relaxed, he will be less allergic than when he is anxious or depressed. Tranquilizers, however, have dangerous side effects and are usually not effective for treating allergic reactions.

Antihistamine drugs are temporarily effective for relieving hay fever symptoms, but they tend to dry out the mucous membranes and thereby increase the patient's sensitivity to allergens with prolonged use. Patients usually develop resistance to antihistamines after taking them for more than a month or so and find them less and less effective as time goes on. Most antihistamines can have serious side effects and should not be used except for temporary relief of severe symptoms.

There is considerable evidence that acupuncture regulates the body's antigen-antibody reactions and can relieve hay fever and other allergic reactions.

Nasal congestion, discharge, and itching are usually relieved during the first acupuncture treatment, but at least six treatments should be taken to give lasting relief of hay fever symptoms. Some patients return for a series of six treatments each year just before what used to be their hay fever season, but others remain free from hay fever for years after one course of acupuncture treatments.

Electric potentiation or twirling is usually not used with acupuncture at facial points but can be used on needles inserted elsewhere for treatment of hay fever.

The most frequently used points for hay fever treatment are:

Meridian points: Co 4, 19, and 20 · Lu 1 and 9 · GB 20 · SI 36 · St 18 · Br 16, 20, and 23

Auricular points: Lung · Internal Nose · Maxillary Sinus

It is important that people with hay fever have large amounts of Vitamins A, C, and Pantothenate as well as a diet including all the other vitamins and essential minerals. The precise dosage should be determined by physicians.

CHRONIC RHINITIS

Rhinitis is a reaction of the nasal mucosa manifested by edema, sneezing, itching, and increased mucus secretion. It may be caused by allergy, usually to a specific antigen, by bacterial infection, or by psychosomatic factors. Treatment involves determination of the specific causative factors. The allergic form of rhinitis may be treated by avoidance of the causative agent or by desensitization with injections of the specific antigen. Desensitizing injections, however, may cause serious adverse reactions or be ineffective. Infections should be treated with antibiotics.

Drug treatment of rhinitis includes the use of vasoconstricting nose drops such as ephedrine, Privine, and Neo-Synephrine. These drugs may give temporary relief but may further irritate the mucous membrane, prolong the symptoms of rhinitis, and may increase susceptibility to nasal and sinus infection.

The acupuncture points for treating chronic rhinitis are:

Meridian points: Co 4, 19, and 20 · GB 20 · Br 16, 20 and 23

The following points should be added for treating atrophic rhinitis:

Meridian points: Co 11 · Sp 6 · SI 36

Auricular points: Internal Nose · Maxillary Sinus

Nasal congestion will usually be relieved and free breathing restored during the first treatment by the time the needles have been in place for 15 minutes. The needles should be left in place for at least 20 minutes, however, and acupuncture repeated at least six times to give lasting relief of symptoms. Electric and heat potentiation are usually unnecessary.

CHRONIC SINUSITIS

The symptoms of chronic sinusitis include headache of a constant or recurrent type, postnasal discharge, sinus pain, vertigo, photophobia, tenderness, and sometimes swelling over the involved sinus. Pain may be localized to the supraorbital region in frontal sinusitis and the upper teeth or cheek in maxillary sinusitis. Sphenoid or ethmoid involvement commonly causes pain in the occipital and parietal regions of the head, behind the nose and eyes, or in the neck. Serous, mucoid, or purulent discharges may be noted on the turbinates or near the ostia of the involved sinuses. Chronic sinusitis is often caused or aggravated by allergies. Acupuncture can relieve these along with the symptoms of sinusitis.

Treatment with nose drops may promote drainage but should be avoided because it may damage the mucosa and extend the infection. Lavage of the involved sinus also may offer temporary relief but extend the infection. Antihistamine drugs remove normal moisture from the mucous membranes and thereby increase the chance of infection. Most antihistamines cause drowsiness and make driving dangerous. Those containing ephedrine cause nervousness, insomnia, and palpitation of the heart.

Acupuncture can usually relieve nasal congestion during the first treatment, but at least four treatments should be given for lasting relief.

Acupuncture points for treating chronic sinusitis are as follows:

Meridian points: Lu 9 · Co 4, 19, and 20 · SI 2 and 36 · GB 20 ·
Me 22 · UB 10 · St 36 · Br 14, 16, 20, and 23

Auricular points: Internal Nose · Maxillary Sinus

No needles should be inserted near an inflamed sinus. The needles on the face should be inserted very superficially over areas which are completely free from signs of inflammation or tenderness.

Acupuncture needles should never penetrate the sinuses or the orbit. Points for treating allergies, depression, and insomnia should be added if these problems seem to be complicating the sinusitis. Electro-potentiation and heat may be helpful and reduce the number of treatments needed for lasting relief. Even if the symptoms are relieved after the first or second treatment, at least four treatments should be given. Some cases of long-standing sinusitis involving headaches and allergies may require ten or more treatments.

Acute sinusitis should be treated with antibiotics rather than with acupuncture, but acupuncture may be used to give almost immediate relief from nasal congestion.

chapter 15

CIRCULATORY DISORDERS

Acupuncture should not be used to treat heart disease, varicose veins, aneurysms, or most other disorders of the cardiovascular system, but it may be effective for relieving the pain of ischemic disorders, such as angina pectoris, Buerger's disease and Raynaud's syndrome. There is some indication that it may also improve the general physiology of ischemic areas.

The regulatory effects of acupuncture tend to reduce hypertension and edema. Antihypertensive and diuretic drugs, however, should not be discontinued except under the close supervision of a physician who decides they are no longer necessary.

HYPERTENSION (HIGH BLOOD PRESSURE)

High blood pressure is a serious condition which can cause heart attacks, strokes, and kidney damage. Since it is a painless condition, many people do not realize they have it until it is discovered during a routine physical examination.

There are many possible causes of hypertension which should be investigated and reduced as much as possible. Drugs which increase urinary output, thereby reducing edema, are effective in lowering blood pressure in many cases but may have undesirable side effects. Tranquilizing drugs reduce blood pressure but cause impaired coordination, drowsiness, and depression or even more serious side effects in many cases. Such drugs, however, should not be discontinued without medical supervision.

Acupuncture is effective in reducing blood pressure in most cases and can be used along with antihypertensive drugs or as a substitute for them in some cases.

Salt and salty foods should be eliminated from the diet. Vitamin E (400 units daily) should be taken to prevent thrombosis and Vitamin C (2 gm. daily) to prevent hemorrhage, along with a diet free from fried and fatty foods, sweets, caffeine, and alcohol. Mild exercise may be beneficial in keeping blood pressure under control, but strenuous exercise may cause heart attacks or strokes if blood pressure is high.

Classical acupuncture points for treating hypertension include:

Meridian points: SI 14 · UB 11 · GB 20 and 21 · Li 13 and 14 · Sx 5 and 15

Auricular points: Kidney · Genitalia · Sympathy · Gonads

EDEMA

Edema is the excessive accumulation of serous fluid in body tissues. Before attempting to relieve this symptom, it is essential to identify its cause since edema may precede pain as a warning of serious disease which requires prompt treatment.

Edema of one leg may be caused by thrombophlebitis, which should not be treated by acupuncture.

The most common causes of symmetrical edema are malfunctions of the heart, kidneys, or liver. Electrocardiograms, urinalyses, and various other laboratory tests should be performed to evaluate the condition of these organs before acupuncture is given.

Parasitic infestations, such as trichinosis or filariasis, may cause edema in various parts of the body and should be treated by appropriate medications. Cortisone and its derivatives given for arthritis or allergies are a frequent cause of edema in the United States but cannot safely be discontinued abruptly. Other drugs and substances causing edema should be eliminated promptly.

The edema from acute allergic reactions can be potentially fatal and usually requires intensive medical treatment as well as elimination of the allergen. This type of edema should not be treated by acupuncture unless more appropriate treatment is not available. In cases of chronic angioneurotic edema, however, acupuncture is safer and sometimes more effective than antihistamines.

The ankle edema from chronic heart disease is usually effectively treated by diuretic drugs, but these sometimes have undesirable side effects. In some cases acupuncture can be more effective than drugs and can be used to potentiate or even replace them. Acupuncture should not, however, be used as a substitute for digitalization of people with chronic heart disease.

Eating too much salt or too little protein will aggravate most types of edema. Except in certain kinds of kidney disease and allergic conditions, anyone with edema should be on a low-salt, high-protein diet which includes essential vitamins and minerals. Tight garments which push edema from one part of the body to another generally interfere with circulation and should be avoided. Elevating the legs may relieve edema temporarily in the ankles, but the surplus fluid will tend to accumulate in the part of the body which is in the lowest position. Raising the foot of the bed, for instance, may result in lung edema, which is more serious than ankle edema.

Chronic edema can often be relieved for many months or years by a series of six acupuncture treatments. Patients should understand, however, that being free from edema does not necessarily mean that they are free from the disease which caused it. They should continue whatever other medical treatment may be indicated.

The classical acupuncture points for treating edema include:

Meridian points: Lu 7 · Co 4 and 6 · Sp 6 and 9 · UB 20, 23, 28, and 39 · Br 4 · St 36

Auricular points: Kidney · Heart · Liver · Abdomen · Shenmen · Urinary Bladder

ISCHEMIC DISORDERS

Angina Pectoris

Pain and a feeling of constriction in the chest from cardiac ischemia can sometimes be relieved by acupuncture but should also be treated with oxygen inhalation, sublingual nitroglycerine tablets (which patients should carry with them at all times), rest, proper diet, digitalis preparations, vasodilators, and diuretics when indicated. Anyone with angina or constricting chest pain should be under the care of a cardiologist who can evaluate his heart condition and determine the medication and amount of exercise he should have.

In many cases, the number of anginal attacks of pain can be reduced and exercise tolerance increased if acupuncture is given along with other appropriate treatment. The anxiety, depression, and insomnia which accompany angina can also be reduced by acupuncture. The points for treating these are given elsewhere in this book.

Treatments can be given on a daily basis for six to ten days or a weekly basis. Usually the angina will be greatly reduced for several months after acupuncture treatment, but another series of acupuncture treatments may be required later to control the pain. There is considerable evidence that acupuncture can lower blood cholesterol levels and thereby reduce the arteriosclerotic process which causes ischemia, angina, and the narrowing of arteries. Taking Vitamin E (d-alphatocopherol, at least 400 International Units daily), Niacinamide (1500 mg.), Vitamin C (2000 mg.), other essential vitamins and minerals as well as lecithin and a low cholesterol, low fat, low sugar, and high protein diet also improves the patient's health and tends to retard the arteriosclerotic process. Since Vitamin E potentiates the effects of anticoagulant drugs, it should not be taken without consulting a physician.

Usually not more than 6–10 points at a time should be used to treat angina pectoris. The points most likely to be effective are:

Meridian points: Me 4 and 6 · Co 4 and 11 · Sp 17 · St 3, 6, and 36 · Br 14 and 20 · UB 13, 20, and 24 · Lu 1 and 7 · Sx 9, 12, 17, and 22 · Va 6 · Li 3 and 10 · Ki 6 and 7 · GB 20

Auricular points: Lung · Heart · Liver · Gall Bladder · Pancreas · Sympathy

Buerger's Disease

Buerger's disease is a progressive inflammatory disorder of the blood vessels, mainly in the legs. Its cause is unknown, but it is aggravated by smoking tobacco and is seldom seen in people who have never smoked. It causes severe pain, can be seriously disabling, and can lead to gangrene requiring amputation.

No antibiotics have been found effective for treating the inflammation of the walls of arteries and veins. Anticoagulants are not considered helpful for reducing thrombus formation in this disease. Vascular surgery is not practicable because most of the blood vessels involved are too small.

Onset of symptoms may be gradual or sudden. Coldness, numbness, tingling, or burning pain in the feet and legs are usually noticed first. The feet may become reddish-purple when in a dependent position but very pale when elevated above the level of the heart. Walking may become extremely painful. Exposure to cold temperatures makes the symptoms worse, and most people with this disease feel better in a warm climate. Any slight injury to the feet or legs tends to become infected and enlarged. If gangrene develops, amputation is usually required.

Acupuncture can relieve the early symptoms of Buerger's disease and retard its progression. Pain is usually significantly relieved after the first few treatments. Circulation begins to improve, and the patient may have months or even years of remission of all symptoms after six to ten treatments. Some patients require a few treatments every month or two to remain in a state of remission. Even long-standing cases of Buerger's disease have been greatly improved by acupuncture. Treatment for smoking addiction can be given at the same time and is usually successful.

Large doses of Vitamin C (5–15 gm. daily) and Vitamin E (400–1200 International Units daily) are helpful and should be taken during and after acupuncture. Vitamin E, however, should not be taken by people on anticoagulant drugs. Other nutrients recommended include Vitamin A (10,000 International Units), B1 (25 mg.), B2 (25 Mg.), Niacin or Niacinamide (1–3 gm.), Pantothenate (100 mg.), Para-aminobenzoic acid (200 mg.), Calcium (100–300 mg.), Magnesium (100 mg.), and Selenium (25 mcg.).

Exercise should be gradually increased as pain is relieved but should not be attempted when thrombophlebitis is present.

Acupuncture points for Buerger's disease include:

Meridian points: St 25, 29, and 30 · Sp 14 and 15 · GB 26 · Va 4 and 5 · Me 5, 6, and 7 · Sx 5 and 6

Auricular points: Ankle · Toes · Gall Bladder · Colon · Liver · Knee · Sympathy

Raynaud's Syndrome

Raynaud's phenomenon, disease, or syndrome is a circulatory disorder characterized by episodes of ischemia in the fingers, and occasionally the toes. These episodes are usually triggered by exposure to cold or emotional trauma, sometimes both. Most cases are ideopathic and relieved by relaxation in a warm atmosphere.

At the onset of an attack, the skin of the fingers and toes becomes extremely pale. Then the involved digits become painful and cyanotic.

People with this disorder have such an intolerance of cold weather that they move to a warm climate if possible. Young people, especially women, may have ideopathic Raynaud's syndrome.

Raynaud's syndrome is more serious when it is secondary to such conditions as occlusive arterial disease, connective tissue disorders, neurogenic lesions, dysproteinemias, ergot or methysergide intoxication, pulmonary hypertension, or trauma. In such cases, the underlying pathology should be treated before acupuncture is used for treatment.

Six acupuncture treatments are usually enough to give relief from ideopathic Raynaud's syndrome for at least a year. Treating cases secondary to severe organic pathology usually requires much longer.

The points for treatment include:

Meridian points: Co 3, 4, and 11 · He 4 and 7 · Lu 3 and 8 · St 36 and 39 · GB 33 · Sp 6

Auricular points: Fingers · Toes · Ankle · Sympathy · Shenmen

chapter 16

DERMATOLOGIC DISORDERS

Skin disorders should be carefully diagnosed and given the benefit of standard treatment before acupuncture is used. Acupuncture may be used to relieve the itching of acute skin disorders but is generally reserved for treatment of chronic skin conditions. Response to acupuncture is often slow. It may require at least ten or more treatments.

Acupuncture needles should never be inserted within skin lesions. The needles should be placed as far from the lesions as possible to avoid spreading them.

The classical points for treating skin disorders include:

Meridian points: Lu 3 and 5 · Co 4, 11, and 16 · St 36 · Sp 10 and 20 · UB 12, 13, 54, and 57 · Ki 26 · GB 30, 31, 35, 38, and 39 · Br 14

Auricular points: Liver · Kidney · Colon · Small Intestine

Allergens which may be causing or aggravating skin lesions should be eliminated as much as possible, and attention should be given to improving nutrition with vitamin and mineral supplements as indicated.

Contact dermatitis may appear as various types of rashes or skin lesions. Acupuncture will promote healing, but the allergen should be identified and avoided if possible.

Urticaria, or *hives*, is usually a reaction to something ingested or injected. If a person continues to take a drug which has given him this type of skin reaction, *angioneurotic edema* or even anaphylactic shock may develop. Acupuncture may relieve the symptoms of such serious disorders somewhat but should not be depended on as the only treatment for anaphylactic shock. Epinephrine and other appropriate medications should be given.

ECZEMA

Eczema is a diagnostic term physicians use for a chronic skin disorder from an unidentified cause. Because of the difficulty in determining the specific cause of many chronic skin diseases, these diseases are called eczema instead of receiving a more precise diagnosis, such as "contact dermatitis," "atopic dermatitis," or "determatitis medicamentosa."

Skin disorders not caused by a specific bacterium or virus are produced and perpetuated by allergic, metabolic, and emotional factors which may be potentiating each other. Medications are the most common allergens in the United States. Even antihistamines given as treatment for respiratory allergies can cause allergic skin reactions. Cortisone derivatives, included in frequently prescribed ointments, can aggravate and delay healing of dermatitis or eczema.

Acupuncture is a safe and effective treatment for eczema because it can reduce allergic reactions, improve body physiology, and relieve such emotional problems as depression, anxiety, and insomnia. Usually six to ten treatments are adequate. Healing should continue after the treatments are completed. Points for treatment include

Meridian points: Co 11 · Sp 10 · UB 12, 13, 54, and 57 · GB 20, 30, 31, 38, and 39 · Br 14

Auricular points: Elbow · Knee · Abdomen · Sympathy

Medications should be discontinued under medical supervision, and an attempt to identify food and other allergens should be made.

Nutrients which are especially helpful in healing eczema are Vitamin A (20,000 units), Vitamin C (2 gm), and Pantothenic acid (200 mg.) daily.

ACNE ROSACEA

Acne rosacea is a reddening and irregular thickening of facial skin, especially on the nose. It is often associated with alcoholism and is, therefore, very embarrassing. Many people with this condition have never drunk alcohol and feel resentful about being falsely accused. Drinking excessive amounts of tea and coffee is also thought to promote this condition for reasons not clearly understood.

By balancing the distribution of body energy, acupuncture can usually reduce the facial redness and the subcutaneous nodules which enlarge the nose and give it a bulbous appearance.

The main acupuncture points for treating acne rosacea are:

Meridian points: UB 1 and 40 · Sp 6 and 10 · Co 4 and 11 · St 1 · Lu 7 · GB 20 and 37

Auricular points: Liver · Kidney

Needles should be inserted superficially at these points and left in place for about 20 minutes. Electropotentiation of 30–50 microamperes can be used. Ten treatments without more than a week between any two of them constitutes a course of treatment. Some signs of improvement should be noted during the first course of treatment and in the month following treatment. Since this is a chronic condition which may respond slowly, several courses of treatment at least a month apart may be required.

ACNE VULGARIS

Acne is a common skin disorder, mostly on the face, neck, and back, which is usually associated with adolescence. Various ointments, lotions, soaps, and diets are helpful in many cases. Recovery is usually spontaneous before age 25. But many cases of acne are resistant and persist beyond puberty, often leaving scars. Antibiotics, such as tetracycline, are useful when the pustules become infected but will not prevent new pimples from appearing. X-ray treatments are effective but cause loss of subcutaneous tissue and even cancer of the face many years after treatment.

Acupuncture can be an effective treatment of acne because of its ability to promote homeostasis and regulate hormone production. It can also combat the depression and other emotional disturbances which often accompany acne.

There is considerable evidence that many American adolescents select a diet which is deficient in vitamins and which contains excessive amounts of refined sugar and fat. During this period of growth and development, it is especially important that people with acne eat a diet high in proteins and low in fat and refined sugar. Vitamins and minerals important for healing acne and promoting good general health are: Zinc sulfate (30 mg.), Vitamin A (20,000 International Units), Vitamin B1 (Thiamin, 20 mg.), Vitamin B2 (Riboflavin, 20 mg.), Vitamin B6 (Pyridoxine, 20 mg.), Niacinamide (1000 mg.), Pantothenate (200 mg.), Vitamin C (2000 mg.), Vitamin D (800 International Units), Vitamin E (d-alphatocopherol, 800 International Units daily). Vitamin E, however, should not be taken by people on anticoagulant drugs. Some good multivitamin products are available to avoid swallowing too many pills each day. The above should be taken along with acupuncture treatments and continued indefinitely afterwards.

Acupuncture points for treating acne are:

Meridian points: Lu 3 and 5 · Co 4, 11, and 16 · Sp 20 · Ki 26 · St 36 · GB 35

Auricular points: Gonads · Liver · External Nose · Spleen · Stomach · Shenmen

Treatments can be given on a daily or weekly basis. Sometimes ten treatments are enough to reverse the acne condition, and healing will be almost completed during the month following treatment. In other cases it is necessary to have another series of ten treatments at least a month after the first.

PSORIASIS

Psoriasis is a chronic inflammatory skin disease characterized by red patches covered with silvery-white scales. It affects mostly the extensor surfaces of the body and the scalp. Although the cause of psoriasis has not been clearly determined, metabolic, climatic, and emotional factors may affect its course.

Medications prescribed for it may have serious side effects and give only temporary relief if any. Exposure of the skin to sunshine and ingestion of large doses of Vitamins C and E are helpful in many cases. Since people with psoriasis usually have elevated cholesterol levels in their blood, a diet to reduce cholesterol is advisable.

Acupuncture has been very effective in treating psoriasis, but many treatments are usually required. Some patients need a series of ten treatments three or four times a year. We advise patients to return for more treatments if the lesions begin to recur, but in some cases this has not been necessary.

Since emotional problems can produce an exacerbation of psoriasis, psychotherapy may be beneficial. Freedom from stress is important for recovery from psoriasis. Acupuncture can also be used to relieve symptoms of anxiety, depression, insomnia, and itching. Allergens affecting psoriasis should be identified if possible and avoided. Acupuncture can reduce allergic reactions.

Acupuncture points within skin lesions should not be used. Points for treating psoriasis include:

Meridian points: Co 4, 11, and 15 · St 36 · Sp 6 and 10 · UB 6, 12, 54, and 60 · Va 3 · GB 20, 30, 31, 38, and 39 · Br 20

Auricular points: Liver · Kidney · Knee · Elbow · Ankle · Spleen · Buttocks · Shenmen

PRURITUS (ITCHING)

Pruritus is an itching sensation, which may be generalized or localized. If localized, the skin should be carefully examined to rule out scabies, pediculosis, insect bites, contact dermatitis, and other causes of a rash. Itching of the anal region may be from pinworms. Generalized pruritus may be a symptom of a systemic disease for which standard American treatment is available. Diabetes mellitus, nephritis, cirrhosis of the liver, carcinoma, leukemia, Hodgkin's disease and thyroid dysfunction may cause pruritus. It is important to rule out all of the above causes of pruritus or be sure that the patient has been given appropriate standard treatment for them before acupuncture is attempted.

Pruritus of allergic or psychogenic etiology may be effectively treated by acupuncture using the following points:

Meridian points: Co 11 · Sp 10 · UB 12, 13, 54, and 57 · GB 20 · Br 14

Auricular points: Liver · Kidney · Shenmen

The itching is usually relieved while the needles are in place for 20 minutes. In most cases, however, acupuncture should be repeated on the following day to ensure lasting relief of the itching. Some cases require six or more treatments.

ALOPECIA (BALDNESS)

Alopecia is hair loss from various causes, which should be determined before treatment is prescribed. Scalp infections and parasitic infestations should be treated with appropriate drugs. Most alopecia or baldness, however, is considered to be of emotional, hormonal, or unknown etiology.

Alopecia areata is characterized by patches of baldness asymmetrically located on the head and caused by emotional reactions. Sometimes the hair grows back spontaneously without treatment, but other bald spots are likely to appear from time to time after an emotional upset. No drugs are useful for treating this type of baldness, but acupuncture can accelerate the regrowth of hair and can usually prevent new bald spots from developing.

The most common type of alopecia or baldness is the asymmetrical hair loss on the top of the head, most common in men but also occurring in some women. It is generally agreed that drugs are ineffective for this condition although many have been recommended.

Acupuncture has been found effective for retarding hair loss and promoting new hair growth in this type of alopecia. A course of six treatments on a daily, or at least weekly, basis should be given and followed by treatments every two months until hair distribution appears normal. This may take six months or longer. There has been only about a 30% success rate in treating alopecia with acupuncture. Since alopecia does not prevent a person from enjoying good health, most people would rather tolerate it than spend time and money on acupuncture treatments.

The acupuncture points for treating alopecia are as follows:

Meridian points: Br 14 · Co 11 · Va 6 · Ki 1 and 3 · UB 23 and 40 · Li 2, 13, and 14 · Sp 10 · GB 20

Auricular points: Liver · Gonads · Pancreas · Kidney

HYPERHIDROSIS (EXCESSIVE PERSPIRATION)

Hyperhidrosis is excessive sweating. People normally sweat or perspire as the body attempts to maintain its temperature in overly warm environments or as metabolism is increased by exercise. Some women perspire so much after menopausal hot flashes that their clothing becomes wet. Many people perspire in response to nervous tension or fear. There is considerable variation in the normal amount of perspiration a person produces in response to various situations. Some people, however, perspire excessively no matter what the temperature of their environment is or how quiet and relaxed they are. These people have the problem of hyperhidrosis, which may be embarrassing and give them an unpleasant body odor.

The main points for acupuncture treatment of hyperhidrosis include:

Meridian points: Co 4 and 11 · Ki 7 · St 36 · Sp 4 · GB 21 · Li 3 · Sx 6 · Br 14 and 20

Auricular points: Kidney · Liver · Forehead · Pancreas · Brain

Six treatments are usually enough to reduce perspiration significantly.

WRINKLES

The condition of the skin and structures beneath it depend on health. People could retain youthful appearance and vigor much longer if their bodies, including all their vital organs, had the correct balance of *Yin-Yang* energy.

Yin energy may be compared with negatively charged electricity and *Yang* with positively charged electricity. Acupuncture theory is based on the body energy system. The acupuncture meridians are the main pathways of energy with a "telephone network" of wires (nerve fibers) for communication; the body energy system can be compared with a radio network that does not need wires for communication. In this analogy, the acupuncture points are broadcasting stations that send messages to adjust the *Yin-Yang* energy balance in various parts of the body for optimal health, as explained in Chapter 4.

Although American doctors have been reluctant to accept the existence of the body energy system, they use this concept whenever they do an electrocardiogram or electroencephalogram.

Imbalances of *Yin-Yang* energy in various parts of the body may be caused by malnutrition, injury, bacterial invasion, drugs, air and water pollution, lack of exercise, and other factors. Nutritional therapy should be used along with acupuncture. Antibiotics should be given if necessary to treat infections, but all tranquilizers and other chemicals which damage the brain and other body organs should be avoided.

Acupuncture treatments for achieving and maintaining the correct *Yin–Yang* energy balance in all parts of the body can restore body function and eliminate the unnecessary outward signs of aging, such as wrinkled skin and sagging muscles.

Considerable improvement in appearance and vitality is usually evident by the time six acupuncture treatments have been given. People who keep their *Yin–Yang* energy in proper balance may look and feel as much as 20 years younger than other people their age.

Acupuncture points for improving facial muscle tone include:

Meridian points: Co 11 · St 2, 4, 6, and 37 · Sp 4 · He 7 · Ki 1 and 3 · Li 2 · Sx 24 · Br 16 and 25

Auricular points: Eye I and II · Gonads · Liver · Kidney · Neck · Forehead · External Nose · Genitalia · Stomach · Colon

chapter 17

GASTRO–INTESTINAL DISORDERS

The gastro-intestinal system can be involved in a number of non-malignant disease processes, including peptic ulceration, constipation, diarrhea, malabsorption, esophageal disorders, nausea, vomiting, appendicitis, regional ileitis, and gall bladder pathology. In many cases, the origin of the abnormal function cannot be elucidated even by extensive medical investigation and is probably psychogenic. The severity of these processes may vary from inconsequential "heartburn" to life-threatening gastric hemorrhage. Even though the cause of digestive disturbances might be emotional, there usually is demonstrable somatic pathology and abnormality of enzyme and acid contents of digestive secretions. Acupuncture may relieve the symptoms of digestive disorders which are not caused by malignancy, parasites, bacteria, perforation of a visceral organ, or mechanical obstruction.

Peptic ulcer disease involves abnormal digestion of the gastro-intestinal mucosa by the normally present hydrochloric acid and proteolytic enzymes. This can be considered a *Yang* condition. Overproduction of acid, or defective mucosal defense mechanisms, are involved in peptic ulceration. Traditional medical treatment is directed toward neutralization of acid with controlled diet and antacids along with anticholinergic therapy. Tagamet is an effective drug for healing peptic ulcers. It should be prescribed along with acupuncture. Vitamin C (2 gms.) daily will decrease the danger of hemorrhage. Acupuncture can reduce the pain and improve physiologic function.

The classical acupuncture points for this are:

Meridian points: St 36, 37, and 44 · UB 10, 11, 17, 18, 21, and 22 · GB 20 · Sp 4

Heat and electropotentiation is usually unnecessary. Some of the points should be used bilaterally, but not all points should be used for each treatment. Usually six treatments will give lasting relief of symptoms.

Diarrheal disorders include allergic reactions, ulcerative colitis, regional enteritis (Crohn's Disease), bacterial infections, parasitic infestations, hepatobiliary disease, and pancreatic malfunction. Severe nervous stress may also be involved in the etiology of diarrhea, as well as in nausea and vomiting. Stool examination should reveal parasites, pathogenic bacteria, blood, and excessive mucus when present. Sigmoidoscopy, cholecystogram, and barium fluroscopy studies of the digestive tract should reveal tumors, strictures, and gallstones.

Acupuncture should not be used to treat bacterial infections, parasitic infestations, tumors, or gall stones, but may be effective in treating diarrheal disorders after these conditions have been ruled out. Stomach cramps, nausea, "heartburn," and flatulence also respond well to acupuncture. If food allergy is suspected, the food should be eliminated if possible and acupuncture points for treating allergies should be added.

Acupuncture points for relieving symptoms of indigestion, diarrhea, and colitis are:

Meridian points: Va 6 · St 25, 36, 37, and 44 · Sx 10, 12, 13, 14, 17 · UB 17–23, and 25 · Co 3 and 4 · Sp 3, 4, and 5 · GB 20 · Li 2, 3, and 12

Auricular points: Pancreas · Abdomen · Colon · Small Intestine

(See also the discussions of Abdominal Pain, Colitis, and Indigestion.)

Heat and electropotentiation may be helpful but are not necessary. Only about 8–12 needles should be inserted for each treatment. Significant improvement should be noticed by the eighth treatment, but more may be needed to give lasting relief.

Constipation can be relieved by acupuncture but should also be treated by increasing fluid intake, especially fruit juices, such as orange, prune, and grape. Adding bran and more green vegetables to the diet may be helpful, especially if diverticulitis is a complication. (See the section on Constipation.)

ABDOMINAL PAIN

Acute abdominal pain is often a warning of serious illness which requires prompt surgical intervention. Appendicitis, cholecystitis, regional ileitis, mesenteric thrombosis, pancreatitis, perforated peptic ulcer, and various other life-threatening conditions produce severe abdominal pain which should not be relieved by analgesics or acupuncture until diagnosis has been made.

Post-surgical abdominal pain caused by intestinal distension, manipulation of viscera during surgery, or the incision can usually be effectively relieved by acupuncture at:

Meridian points: Co 4 • St 25, 36, and 40 • Va 6 • UB 25 • Me 6 • Li 3 • Sx 6 and 14

Auricular points: Stomach • Small Intestine • Liver • Pancreas • Colon • Shenmen

The needles can be twirled or left in place 20 minutes, and the procedure can be repeated every four hours if necessary.

Chronic abdominal pain which has been adequately diagnosed can be relieved by acupuncture while other appropriate treatment of the condition causing the pain is being given. Even the severe pain of terminal cancer can usually be relieved by acupuncture, but acupuncture should not be used as a substitute for other treatment of cancer.

Pain from ulcerative colitis, diverticulitis, peptic ulcer, or adhesions can often be relieved by acupuncture if the patient is observed carefully for symptoms of perforation, hemorrhage, or intestinal obstruction requiring surgical intervention. Acupuncture seems to promote homeostasis and a feeling of well-being which is generally beneficial to all conditions with a psychosomatic component.

Undiagnosed chronic abdominal pain should not be treated by acupuncture unless all appropriate diagnostic procedures have been performed with negative results and psychogenic etiology seems most likely. In such cases, acupuncture is advisable along with careful observation of the patient to rule out symptoms of serious complications.

Six to ten acupuncture treatments given on a daily, or at least a weekly, basis should be sufficient to give lasting relief from non-specific abdominal pain. Treatment of ulcerative colitis usually takes longer and should be accompanied by a diet free from alcohol, drugs, spicy foods, and suspected allergens. Patients with colitis often suffer from malnutrition and generally benefit from a high protein diet supplemented by vitamins. (See Chapter 7.)

The acupuncture points most frequently used for treating chronic abdominal pain are:

Meridian points: Co 4 and 11 · UB 18 · St 36 · Va 6 · Li 3 · Sp 4 · He 7

Auricular points: Stomach · Small Intestine · Liver · Pancreas · Colon · Shenmen

COLITIS

Colitis is inflammation and malfunction of the colon. There are two basic types of colitis—ulcerative and spastic.

Ulcerative colitis is much more serious and is characterized by the frequent passage of bloody stools. Its cause is known, but its onset is usually associated with emotional stress and frustration. Antibiotics and cortisone derivatives may relieve symptoms of inflammation temporarily, but antibiotics may cause allergic reactions or encourage the growth of fungi while corticoids may increase the danger of perforation. Some cases of ulcerative colitis remain chronic for many years with brief periods of remission, but others become rapidly so severe that surgical removal of the colon is necessary.

Spastic colitis is considered mainly a functional disorder and is much less serious but sometimes very persistent. It is characterized by diarrhea with mucus excretion alternating with episodes of constipation. Taking laxatives aggravates the condition and should be avoided. Laxatives, such as cascara, irritate the intestines and are not helpful. Sedatives promote constipation. There is no known drug which is effective for treating this condition, but a high fiber diet with plenty of liquids and all the essential vitamins is beneficial. Large doses of Vitamin C will help prevent bleeding.

Physicians should prescribe appropriate diets and nutritional supplements for patients with colitis to take during and after acupuncture therapy. They can also give psychotherapy or personal counseling.

Patients who have been taking ACTH or cortisone derivatives for colitis should not discontinue their drugs suddenly because withdrawal symptoms can be life-threatening. Physicians must supervise the gradual reduction of these dangerous drugs.

Acupuncture is effective for treating both types of colitis. Six treatments are usually enough for lasting relief from spastic colitis, but ulcerative colitis may require many more treatments. Acupuncture can also be used to treat anxiety and depression which frequently accompany and aggravate colitis. Most patients experience a feeling of well-being after the first few treatments.

Classical points for treating colitis include:

Meridian points: Co 3 and 4 · St 25, 36, 37, and 44 · Sp 3, 4, 6, and 15 · UB 17, 18, 19, 21, 22, 23, and 25 · Li 2, 3, and 12 · Sx 6, 10, 12, 13, 14, and 17 · GB 20 · Va 6

Auricular points: Abdomen · Colon · Pancreas · Small Intestine

CONSTIPATION

Although few people have a bowel movement at the same time each day, many people consider themselves constipated because they don't. These people injure their intestines by taking laxatives. Drug companies give dangerous misinformation in their laxative advertising and encourage people to worry needlessly about constipation and to take drugs which are harmful and less effective than safer treatment.

Acupuncture is usually effective for relieving constipation by improving body physiology. Six treatments is usually enough, even if a patient has suffered from constipation for many years.

Along with acupuncture, a patient should drink several glasses of fruit juice a day. Since citrus juice in such large quantities may cause mild bladder irritation, unsweetened grape, prune, or fig juice can be used. Increasing water intake is also helpful. To restore and maintain the intestines in good condition, foods containing fiber should be included in the diet. Raw vegetables, bran, whole wheat, oats, sunflower seeds, and many fruits are good sources of fiber. Cheese, milk, eggs, and meat in the diet should be reduced to avoid constipation, although they are of nutritional value.

Lack of exercise, depression, resentment, repressed hostility, and excessive concern with neatness and cleanliness may cause constipation. Increasing exercise and enjoyment of life in general will tend to discourage constipation.

The main points for treating constipation are:

Meridian points: Co 7 · St 25 and 40 · Sp 3 and 15 · UB 25 · Ki 3 · Me 6 · Sx 6

Auricular points: Sympathy · Pancreas · Colon · Rectum · Liver · Small Intestine

HIATUS HERNIA

Hiatus hernia is the upward movement of part of the stomach through the esophageal opening in the diaphragm. It is a very common condition in people past thirty and may produce pain, discomfort, and shortness of breath mimicking a heart attack.

Surgery to reduce the size of the opening may be somewhat effective in some cases but is dangerous. If the size of the opening is reduced too much, food will have difficulty passing from the esophagus into the stomach. If the opening is not reduced enough, the hiatus hernia will recur. For this reason, most physicians recommend conservative therapy with weight reduction, exercise and avoidance of horizontal posture after eating. Certain drugs, including tranquilizers, antacids, and antispasmodics, may be somewhat effective, but they may produce serious side effects.

Acupuncture is a safe and effective treatment for hiatus hernia. It can be used for weight control and reduction of nervous tension at the same time.

Diet and nutritional therapy can be helpful and are prescribed by physicians at the Washington Acupuncture Center. They may also recommend changes in eating habits and exercises.

Acupuncture points for relieving symptoms include:

Meridian points: Co 11 and 15 · St 25, 26, and 40 · UB 23, 25, and 54 · GB 30 · Me 6 · Li 3 · Sx 6 and 14

Auricular points: Diaphragm · Abdomen · Stomach · Esophagus

HICCUPS

Hiccups are spasms of the diaphragm from irritation of the afferent or efferent nerves for muscles of respiration, especially the diaphragm. It may also be caused by irritation of medullary centers controlling respiration by such toxins as alcohol. Disorders of the stomach, esophagus, intestines, stomach, liver, and mediastinum may also cause hiccups. Most people have brief, self-limiting episodes of hiccups occasionally without significant pathology or distress, but hiccups can be symptoms of serious diseases or persist for hours, days, or even weeks and be very debilitating.

Most cases respond to such simple measures as drinking a glass of water rapidly or breathing into a paper bag. Pressure over the phrenic nerve in the neck may be effective. For persistent hiccups, some physicians inject procaine to block the phrenic nerve or even perform bilateral phrenicotomy.

Acupuncture is usually effective for treating persistent hiccups regardless of their cause. The points used include:

Meridian points: Sx 12, 22 · Va 6 · UB 17–21 · SI 14 · GB 24 and 40 · Li 13 · Me 6 · St 25 · Sp 6

Auricular points: Diaphragm · Pharynx · Stomach · Esophagus · Shenmen · Sympathy

ILEUS

A paralysis of intestinal motility following surgery, especially abdominal, is a common complication referred to as "ileus." This may be a manifestation of the intestino-intestinal inhibitory reflex, which produces inhibition of intestinal motor activity as a response to intestinal distention. Paralytic ileus usually resolves spontaneously, but cases of persistent ileus require prolonged intravenous therapy and may interfere with healing in bowel surgery.

The following acupuncture points can be used to facilitate the resolution of ileus:

Meridian points: Co 4 · St 25, 36, and 40 · UB 25 · Me 6 · Li 3 · Sx 6 and 14

Some of these points can be used bilaterally. Auricular points may be used with, instead of, or after the major meridian points. These include Small Intestine · Stomach · Colon · Abdomen · Liver · Pancreas. Heat and electricity are usually not necessary but may be helpful. The needles should be left in place for about 20 minutes or longer if there is a delayed response.

If a patient has been adequately prepared for surgery by fasting and enemas, there should be no danger of intestinal obstruction persistent enough to require more surgery.

INDIGESTION

Any malfunction of the digestive system may be called indigestion and is a common medical problem. It may be caused by contaminated food, emotional distress, malnutrition, hiatus hernia, or allergic reactions. Persistent indigestion may be a symptom of peptic ulcer, gall bladder, liver, pancreas, or kidney disease. If accompanied by severe pain, it may be caused by a serious condition requiring prompt surgery, such as acute appendicitis, mesenteric thrombosis, or regional ileitis.

Medicines advertised for the treatment of indigestion, such as Alka Seltzer, contain aspirin, one of the most common causes of stomach ulcers and internal bleeding. Cortisone also encourages the development of stomach ulcers, although it is frequently prescribed for colitis, allergies, arthritis, and many other medical problems. Most antibiotics and almost every other drug can cause some people to have indigestion. Flatulence, burping, or heartburn are common symptoms of indigestion.

Acupuncture is safer and usually more effective than any drug for treating chronic indigestion. It can also relieve anxiety and depression which may be causative factors. Six to ten treatments are usually required for lasting relief.

Allergenic foods and artificial and biological contaminants should be avoided. Vitamins, especially C and the B complex, should be added to a diet high in proteins, whole grain cereals, fruits, and slightly cooked vegetables.

Acupuncture points for indigestion include:

Meridian points: Co 3 and 4 · St 36 · Sp 4 and 5 · UB 17, 18, and 19 · GB 20 · Va 6 · Sx 14 and 17

Auricular points: Esophagus · Abdomen · Small Intestine · Liver · Pancreas · Colon · Diaphragm

VOMITING

Vomiting as a postsurgical complication may pose a serious hazard, especially in abdominal and thoracic procedures. The use of Compazine, Thorazine, and trimethobenzamide may be contraindicted or ineffective in a specific patient. Acupuncture may be an important modality of treatment in such cases.

The most commonly used points to relieve postsurgical nausea and vomiting are St 36 and Va 6. These points should be used bilaterally. The needles are usually inserted for 20 minutes and not potentiated by heat or electricity. Some of the points for relieving abdominal cramps may also be used. These are:

Meridian points: St 25 and 40 · Me 6 · and Li 3

Auricular points: Esophagus · Stomach · Small Intestine · Liver · Diaphragm · Shenmen · Sympathy

Nausea and vomiting from any cause may be relieved by acupuncture at the above points, but vomiting is not considered undesirable if it results from food poisoning or ingestion of toxic chemicals. Usually this type of vomiting stops when the offensive stomach contents have been expelled. If "dry heaves" persist after the stomach is empty, acupuncture at the above points is helpful. They can also be used to control the nausea and vomiting of seasickness.

chapter 18

GENITAL DISORDERS

The genital problems for which acupuncture might be used effectively include sexual dysfunction (both male and female), amenorrhea, breast hypoplasia, penis hypoplasia, menstrual disorders, infertility, obstetrics, and menopausal syndrome.

SEXUAL DYSFUNCTION

Sexual impotence is usually classified as functional or psychogenic without demonstrable organic pathology. In women, sexual impotence is called "frigidity," "functional dyspareunia," or "inability to achieve orgasm" and is considered a less serious symptom than a man's inability to achieve and sustain penile erection for a normal length of time.

Some men and women take large quantities of sex hormones in an effort to improve their ability to engage in coitus and enjoy it, but these may have the opposite effect and usually decrease fertility. Psychoanalysis and other forms of psychotherapy are sometimes effective but require many hours over a long period of time (sometimes years).

205

Freud's libido theory and Bergson's theory of *elan vital* are consistent with Chinese acupuncture theory in that they attribute sexual impotence to a perversion or displacement of vital energy. Correcting this situation by restoring the balance between *Yin* and *Yang* energy with acupuncture takes much less time and is usually less emotionally painful than psychotherapy, but psychotherapy along with acupuncture may be helpful.

During the first ten treatments, the patient should avoid sexual intercourse. If results are not satisfactory during the following two weeks, another series of ten treatments should be given. More than half of the patients treated for sexual impotence at the Washington Acupuncture Center have had significant improvement after ten treatments.

Tea, coffee, tobacco, alcohol, hormones, tranquilizers, and other drugs may reduce sexual desire or potency and should be avoided. Nutritional therapy along with acupuncture should include daily supplements of zinc sulfate (30 mg.), Vitamin E (d-alphatocopherol, 400 International Units), Vitamin C (3 gm.), Vitamin B1 (25 mg.), B2 (25 mg.), B6 (25 mg.), Niacinamide (1 gm.), Pantothenate (100 mg.), and Biotin (25 mcg.).

Acupuncture points for relieving sexual impotence include:

Meridian points: St 36 · Sp 6 and 9 · UB 23, 32, and 52 · GB 3 · Sx 3 and 4 · Li 8 · Br 4

Auricular points: Gonads · Urethra · Uterus · Genitalia · Lumbar · Brain

AMENORRHEA

Amenorrhea is absence of menstrual periods. Some normal females do not begin menstruating until age 17 and do not menstruate monthly until they are past 20. Usually menstruation continues monthly until a woman is past 40, except during pregnancy and lactation. If a woman does not menstruate at all until she is 18, she should have diagnostic studies to rule out organic abnormalities. Delayed puberty can be the result of zinc deficiency or other nutritional problems which can be easily remedied. Hormone deficiencies are often caused by nutritional deficiencies, and it is safer to prescribe the proper diet with vitamin and mineral supplements than to describe hormones. Structural abnormalities of the reproductive organs may require surgical correction, and tumors of these organs or of the endocrine glands should be removed if present. In most cases, however, delayed puberty can be corrected by nutritional therapy and acupuncture when no structural abnormalities or tumors are present.

Other possible causes of amenorrhea include tuberculosis, anemia, leukemia, lupus erythematosus, mental illness, and medication with such drugs as chlorpromazine. Acupuncture is a safe and effective substitute for psychotropic drugs and can be given to treat mental illness at the same time as amenorrhea. Infectious and malignant diseases, however, should not be treated with acupuncture until other appropriate treatment has been instituted.

It is not necessarily abnormal for a woman to miss a few menstrual periods, and many healthy women in their thirties have an early menopause. In general, amenorrhea is a much less serious symptom than excessive, too frequent, or painful menstruation. Worry about amenorrhea is often more of a problem than the amenorrhea.

Six to ten treatments are usually effective for relieving amenorrhea in women who are free from nutritional deficiencies and organic pathology. The first six treatments should not be more than a week a apart, and acupuncture is usually given bilaterally at some of the following points:

Meridian points: Co 4, 15, and 18 · St 25 and 36 · Sx 3 and 4 · Sp 6, 8, and 10 · Va 6 · Br 14 · UB 11, 18, 21, 31, 32, and 33 · Li 8 · GB 20 · He 6 and 7 · Me 6 and 8 · Lu 2, 5, and 10 · SI 3

Auricular points: Gonads · Uterus · Liver · Spleen · Genitalia

BREAST HYPOPLASIA

Acupuncture has been effective in stimulating breast development in many cases. The desirability of having breasts of more than minimal size, however, is more related to psychology, culture, and fashion than to physical health. Women with small breasts are at least as likely to be able to nurse their babies as are women with large breasts. Childbirth and lactation will usually enlarge the breasts, and they will remain an optimal size afterwards if sudden weaning or tight breast binders are not involved. But many American men are especially attracted to large breasts, and some women are eager to please them.

Women with low self-esteem have submitted to surgical procedures or extremely hazardous silicone injections to have their breasts enlarged. Too many have lost their breasts and even their lives as a result. Millions of dollars have been earned by the sellers of various "exercise" gadgets which are purported to augment breasts but usually diminish their muscular support instead. In general, exercising without wearing a supporting brassiere will tend to make breasts sag and consequently appear smaller.

Female hormone therapy may be effective for enlarging the breasts but may promote cancer, thrombophlebitis, strokes, heart attacks, and other disorders. It is, therefore, not recommended.

Correcting nutritional deficiencies and acupuncture are the safest treatments likely to be effective for breast augmentation. Six to ten acupuncture treatments with a week or less between treatments will usually result in some increase in breast size and firmness if acupuncture is going to be effective. Breast development may continue for as long as three months after the treatments are over.

Emotional and marital problems should be suspected and treated with psychotherapy in most women who seek breast augmentation. Often conjoint therapy with the husband or consort is helpful. Acupuncture points for anxiety and depression can be used along with those for breast augmentation.

The acupuncture points for stimulating breast development include:

Meridian points: Sx 17 · St 19 · He 2 · SI 4 · Co 11

Auricular points: Gonads · Uterus · Liver · Brain

Acupuncture needles should never be inserted into breast tissue.

PENIS HYPOPLASIA

Having a small penis makes many men feel embarrassed and sexually inferior to men with larger penises. There is a prevalent American belief that the larger a man's penis is, the more appreciated he will be as a sexual partner. Although women are generally more concerned with a man's skill in making love and his ability to maintain an erection than with the size of his penis, penis size is closely related to the self-esteem of many American men.

Acupuncture treatments can stimulate penis growth and, in many cases, increase ability to sustain an erection. Acupuncture is much safer for this purpose than hormone injections, which may promote prostate hypertrophy and arteriosclerosis.

Ten acupuncture treatments are usually enough to produce noticeable penis augmentation. Additional growth will usually take place during the month following the treatments. Some men require an additional series of ten treatments to achieve the penis size that seems satisfactory to them.

No acupuncture needles are inserted into the penis, scrotum, or prostate. Some of the needles for this purpose are inserted into the arms, legs, and ears.

The points for promoting penis growth and erectile capacity are:

Meridian points: Lu 3, 4, and 10 · He 4, 6, and 8 · Va 4 and 8 · Sp 3 and 6 · St 36 and 44 · GB 34 and 43 · Sx 5 and 7 · Br 24

Auricular points: Genitalia · Sympathy · Gonads · Buttocks · Brain

Nutritional therapy including zinc should be given along with acupuncture.

MENSTRUAL DISORDERS

Menstrual disorders include amenorrhea (absence of menses), oligomenorrhea (scanty or infrequent menses), dysmenorrhea (painful menses), premenstrual tension, and menometrorrhagia (excessive menstruation). The latter condition is the only one which should not be treated by acupuncture. It may be a symptom of a serious disorder, such as cancer, which requires prompt diagnosis and standard treatment. Any vaginal bleeding after the menopause also requires prompt diagnosis and should not be treated with acupuncture.

Many women have excessive blood loss with menstruation because of using intrauterine contraceptive devices or taking estrogens. Vitamin C deficiency is another cause of excessive bleeding which can be easily corrected.

Acupuncture treatment of amenorrhea, oligomenorrhea, dysmenorrhea, and premenstrual tension includes the following points:

Meridian points: Co 4, 15, and 18 · St 25 and 36 · Sp 6, 8, and 10 · UB 11, 18, 21, 31, 32, and 33 · He 6 and 7 · Me 6 and 8 · Lu 2, 5, and 10 · GB 20 · SI 3 · Sx 3 and 4 · Br 14

Auricular points: Genitalia · Uterus · Urinary Bladder · Abdomen · Shenmen · Sympathy

INFERTILITY

Inability to become a natural parent has many possible causes, some of which can be effectively treated by acupuncture. Before having acupuncture for infertility, a couple should have thorough physical examinations to rule out anatomical causes of infertility. These should be corrected if possible. Unless both partners have the anatomical requirements for reproduction, acupuncture cannot be helpful. Most drugs reduce fertility and should be eliminated if possible.

Acupuncture, along with nutritional treatment, can raise a man's sperm count considerably and make a woman's reproductive organs more receptive to conception and pregnancy. Acupuncture should be discontinued after conception, but the nutritional program should be continued. Acupuncture is the safest anesthesia for childbirth, but it may induce premature labor or abortion if used during gestation.

Masculine fertility may be increased by vitamins of the B Complex, large doses of Vitamin C (2–5 gm. daily), Vitamin E (800 units daily) and zinc sulfate (30–80 mg. daily). Even larger doses of Vitamin C may be required to help a woman maintain a pregnancy if she has a tendency to miscarry. Diet and vitamin supplements should be discussed with physicians and taken in accordance with their prescriptions.

Acupuncture is also an effective treatment for male impotence and female inability to enjoy sexual relations.

Points for treating infertility include:

Meridian points: St 33 · Sp 4 and 8 · UB 23 and 25 · Li 3 and 8 · Sx 2, 3, 4, 5, and 6 · Br 4

Auricular points: Gonads · Uterus · Brain · Lumbar · Liver

OBSTETRICS

There are certain acupuncture points which can be used to initiate labor for childbirth, and acupuncture at these points can also be used for abortion. As in other situations, the skill of the acupuncturist and precise location of points determine whether acupuncture will be effective. It is less dependable but safer than other methods and could be tried before resorting to more traumatic procedures.

The acupuncture points to initiate labor are: Co 4 · St 36 · Sp 6.

Needles should be applied bilaterally and twirled or have electronic instruments attached to produce a current of 50–200 microamperes for at least 20 minutes. This procedure can be repeated every two to three hours.

It is very important to avoid genital contamination, and aseptic technique should be used to avoid infecting the genital area. If excessive bleeding occurs, appropriate medical treatment should be given.

Chapter 13 contains a list of points to use for obstetrical analgesia.

Although the points used for induction of labor or abortion can also be recommended for contraception, acupuncture is probably less dependable than condoms or diaphragms with contraceptive jelly. Acupuncture at the above points may be used by women a few hours before or immediately after intercourse to diminish the chances of conception.

MENOPAUSAL SYNDROME

Hot flashes, and feeling suddenly too warm without a fever or change in environmental temperature are among the unpleasant symptoms many women experience several years before and after the cessation of their menstrual periods. Some women have blushing of the face and neck along with the sensation of unpleasant warmth. They may be further embarrassed by profuse sweating following the hot flash.

Until recently, physicians routinely prescribed estrogens for women past the age of 35 who complained of hot flashes and other symptoms associated with menopause. Unfortunately, many women have had their chances for developing cancer, thrombophlebitis, strokes, and heart attacks greatly increased by this medical practice. Most physicians are now aware of this danger and prescribe psychotropic drugs instead.

Psychotropic drugs, such as Valium, Librium, Thorazine, and Mellaril, apparently do not promote cancer, but there is evidence that they may damage the heart muscle and the brain. These tranquilizers impair coordination and cause drowsiness, making a person incapable of driving a car efficiently. In many cases, they increase depression. The antidepressant drugs, with which the tranquilizers are often combined, are seldom very effective and produce many serious side effects.

Psychotherapy or some type of counseling can be helpful in dealing with a woman's changing life situation as her children leave home and her aging husband worries about sexual impotence. Many women enjoy sex more than ever after menopause because they no longer have to worry about birth control and are freer from household responsibilities. Psychotherapy can be given along with acupuncture and nutritional therapy. To avoid osteoporosis, Vitamin C (2 gm.), Vitamin D (800 International Units), and calcium lactate (2-6 gm.) should be taken daily. Pantothenic acid (200 mg.) and Vitamin E (400 International Units) help relieve hot flashes and prevent strokes and heart attacks. Other vitamins and minerals are also important.

Acupuncture points for treatment of hot flashes include:

Meridian points: Co 11 · St 19, 29, and 30 · Sp 6 and 8 · UB 23 and 25 · SI 1 · He 2 · Li 3 and 8 · Sx 4 and 17

Auricular points: Liver · Kidney · Uterus · Gonads · Genitalia · Brain

chapter 19

MUSCULOSKELETAL DISORDERS

Acupuncture will not change bony abnormalities or restore completely atrophied tissues, but it is useful for relieving pain, stiffness, and swelling of muscles and joint structures. Musculoskeletal disorders amenable to acupuncture treatment are discussed in this chapter. Pain syndromes from muscle disorders are discussed in Chapter 20.

ARTHRITIS

The term *arthritis* means "inflammation of the joints," and usually involves pain, stiffness, and limitation of function. *Rheumatism* is another name for it. Although arthritis occurs in a number of different forms, there are essentially two major types: (1) inflammatory, which may be exudative, proliferative, or a combination of both; and (2) degenerative, which may result from injury, malnutrition, and limited capacity of the articular cartilaginous surface to repair itself. The

213

first group includes the types of arthritis associated with infective agents, rheumatoid arthritis, ankylosing spondylitis, and connective tissue disorders. The second group comprises degenerative joint diseases, such as osteoarthritis and hypertrophic arthritis.

Gout is a form of arthritis characterized by increased blood uric acid and is basically a metabolic disorder. In cases of persistent gouty arthritis, acupuncture can be given along with any prescribed medication to relieve the unpleasant symptoms.

Most types of arthritis tend to be relentlessly progressive, with increasing joint destruction, pain, and limitation of motion. Until the disease becomes severe, many people relieve their symptoms with non-prescription drugs containing aspirin (acetylsalysilic acid). Unfortunately, this tends to cause stomach ulcers and a generalized bleeding tendency. Phenylbutazone and indomethacin may also give temporary relief, but their use is associated with a large number of toxic, and sometimes fatal, side effects. For arthritis that does not respond to the above drugs, some physicians prescribe such toxic substances as gold salts, antimalarial agents, corticosteroids, and immunosuppressive therapy with cytoxan and imuran. The harm these chemicals do to a patient's general health outweighs their temporary advantages.

Megavitamin therapy with high doses of Vitamin C and Pantothenate is helpful in reducing arthritis symptoms and the bleeding induced by many antiarthritis drugs. These vitamins help restore the function of adrenal glands suppressed by cortisone and its derivatives. They should be instituted promptly and continued after acupuncture. Corticoid drugs must be reduced very slowly to avoid serious withdrawal symptoms, but most other antiarthritis drugs can be discontinued as soon as pain is relieved by acupuncture.

The Washington Acupuncture Center has treated over 10,000 patients for various forms of arthritis and more than 80% of them have had significant improvement. (See Chapter 12 for research on acupuncture treatment of arthritis.) Most patients have their pain, swelling, and stiffness significantly relieved by the time they have had six to ten acupuncture treatments. Some of them have remained free from these symptoms for more than five years after their first course of treatments. Others have had a recurrence of pain after a year or six months, but the pain was relieved again after another course of treatment. Some people with severe rheumatoid arthritis have been able to stay almost symptom-free by having maintenance treatments once a week or less often. They have been able to discontinue the corticoids, phenylbutazone, gold salts, and other dangerous drugs they have been taking and have a normal life. Acupuncture will not change bony deformities, of course, but it is remarkable how well a person can function in spite of these if he is free from pain and stiffness.

The classical acupuncture points used for treating all types of arthritis include the following:

General

    Meridian points: Co 4, 10, 11, and 15 · St 36 · Sp 4 · Me 6 · GB 20, 21, 30, 34, and 39 · Br 14

Shoulders

    Meridian points: Co 15 · Me 14 · SI 9

    Auricular points: Elbow · Neck · Sympathy

Spinal

    Meridian points: UB 10–35 · Br 4, 11, and 14

Cervical

    Meridian points: Co 11, 15, and 16 · SI 19 · GB 39

    Auricular points: Neck · Shoulder

Elbows

    Meridian points: Co 10 and 11 · St 36 · GB 21 · Va 3

    Auricular points: Elbow · Shenmen

Wrists and Hands

    Meridian points: Me 4, 5, and 6 · Co 6 and 11 · SI 4 and 7 · He 7 · Va 5 · Sp 10

    Auricular points: Fingers · Shenmen

Thumbs

    Meridian points: Co 4, 5, and 6 · Lu 9, 10, and 11

Index Fingers

    Meridian points: Co 1, 2, and 3 · Va 7 and 8

Middle Fingers

    Meridian points: Va 9 · Me 3

Ring Fingers

    Meridian points: Me 1, 2, and 3 · He 8 · SI 5

Little Fingers

    Meridian points: SI 2 and 3 · He 7 and 8

Hips

    Meridian points: GB 30, 31, and 34 · UB 30, 31, 48, and 49 · St 28–31 · Li 12 · Sp 13

    Auricular points: Hip · Sacral · Coccygeal

Thighs

    Meridian points: GB 30, 31, and 29 · UB 49

    Auricular points: Hip · Sacral · Lumbar · Shenmen

Knees

    Meridian points: St 34, 35, 36, and 41 · UB 54 · GB 34, 39, and 40 · Li 4 and 8 · Sp 9

    Auricular points: Knees · Shenmen

Ankles

    Meridian points: Sp 5 · St 41 · GB 40 · UB 59–62 · Li 4 · Ki 3–8

    Auricular points: Ankle · Shenmen

Toes in general

    Auricular points: Toes · Shenmen

Great toe

    Meridian points: Sp 1, 2, and 3 · Li 1, 2, and 3

Second toe

    Meridian points: Li 2, 3, and 4 · St 43, 44, and 45

Middle toe

    Meridian points: Li 4 · GB 41

Fourth toe

    Meridian points: GB 42, 43, and 44

Little toe

    Meridian points: UB 64, 65, 66, and 67

Gout

    Meridian points: St 36 · GB 34 · Co 8 and 9 · Me 6

    Auricular points: Shenmen · Sympathy · Liver · Kidney · Pancreas · Stomach · Small Intestine

Infrared heat potentiation is usually helpful. Electric potentiation is beneficial at most of these points but should be avoided on the face and with patients who have heart irregularities.

CONNECTIVE TISSUE DISORDERS RELATED TO ARTHRITIS

Some serious connective tissue disorders include arthritis symptoms and are, therefore, thought to be related to arthritis. Like arthritis, they have an obscure etiology which may be similar to that of arthritis. Those which may be helped by acupuncture include lupus erythematosus, polymyositis, Sjögren's syndrome, and Reiter's syndrome.

Lupus erythematosus may be cutaneous or systemic, the latter being much more serious. It may afflict young people, especially women, and progress from the skin to connective tissues throughout the body. The typical skin lesions are circumscribed macules and plaques with erythema, follicular plugging, scales, telangiectasis and atrophy. Sunlight exacerbates the skin lesions. The main medications given to treat lupus are cortisone derivatives and antimalaria drugs. These medications bring only temporary relief of symptoms and may cause other problems. Selection of acupuncture points to treat lupus depends on the symptomology.

Polymyositis is simultaneous inflammation of many muscles. It is a painful and disabling condition which may respond to acupuncture for relief of pain in the afflicted areas.

Reiter's syndrome is urethritis, conjunctivitis, and polyarthritis. Because of the similarity of its symptoms to gonorrheal arthritis, a course of antibiotics should be given before acupuncture. The arthritic manifestations of Reiter's syndrome should be treated with acupuncture points similar to those for treating other types of arthritis.

Sjögren's syndrome is a symptom complex that includes polyarthritis, enlargement of the parotid gland, and drying of the conjunctiva, mucous membranes of the mouth, nasopharynx, and bronchial tree. No medications have been found helpful for treatment of this disorder.

Acupuncture treatment includes points for treating arthritic joints and the following points for improving the physiology of the conjunctiva and mucous membranes:

Meridian points: Co 20 · Lu 7 and 9 · Br 24 and 25 · St 12 and 14
· Ki 20 · GB 33 and 43 · Li 6 · Sp 3

Auricular points: Shenmen · Lung · Pharynx · Internal Nose · Maxillary Sinus · Thoracic

CERVICAL SYNDROMES

Pain, stiffness and muscle spasms of the neck may arise from many different causes. It is important to diagnose the basic cause before acupuncture is attempted and to rule out conditions which would not respond well to acupuncture. Most neck problems, however, can be effectively relieved by acupuncture in six to ten treatments.

Some of the most common causes of neck problems are arthritis and cervical disc pathology. These factors may combine to put pressure on cervical nerves thereby producing painful muscle spasms with stiffness and limitation of movement. Torticollis is a persistent spasm of neck muscles, which usually can be effectively relieved by acupuncture. Whiplash injuries to the neck encourage the development of all these problems or aggravate pre-existing pathology. Even pain and paresthesia of the arms may be caused by neck problems, and headaches may be triggered by them.

Traction and cervical collars may increase, rather than relieve, muscle spasms. Surgery of the neck area is extremely dangerous and may result in paralysis of the rest of the body by damaging the spinal cord. Drugs which relieve neck pain and muscle spasms have serious side effects and should be avoided. None of them has any lasting therapeutic value.

Nutritional therapy may be helpful and can be given along with acupuncture. Physicians can prescribe a specific program.

Acupuncture points for treating pain and stiffness of the neck include:

Meridian points: SI 3 · UB 10, 60, and 62 · GB 20 and 37

Auricular points: Neck · Sympathy

Points for treating torticollis include:

Meridian points: St 9–12 · Co 4, 16, 17, and 18 · Me 14–16 · GB 20 and 21 · UB 10 and 11 · Br 12–14

WHIPLASH RESIDUALS

Whiplash injuries result from sudden overextension of the neck usually caused by automobile accidents. Although X-ray findings are often negative, pains in the neck and headache resulting from such injury may persist for years. Osteoarthritis of the cervical spine may be promoted by whiplash injuries and cause considerable disability. The gross stress reaction from this type of injury can also be disabling.

Aspirin and narcotics can give temporary relief of the pain but should not be taken for more than a few days. "Muscle relaxant" drugs are usually not very effective. Valium is frequently prescribed for relaxation, but it is addictive and has undesirable side effects. Major tranquilizers, such as Thorazine or Mellaril, have even more serious side effects, including damage to the brain and heart. Physiotherapy may be helpful in some cases if skillfully performed.

Acupuncture is generally the most effective and safest treatment for whiplash residuals. It relieves the muscle spasms and pain promptly, often during the first or second treatment. Six treatments are usually enough to give lasting relief, even after arthritis has been demonstrated by X-ray, but in some cases ten or more may be needed.

Many patients with whiplash residuals wear an orthopedic collar, which does more harm than good in most cases. These collars may aggravate muscle spasms and cause the patient to hold his neck in an unnatural position. They may also interfere with blood circulation and put pressure on nerves, thereby increasing pain.

Traction for whiplash injuries may relieve pain temporarily and be harmless if used for less than an hour at a time. Prolonged bedrest with traction, however, may promote hypostatic pneumonia or thrombophlebitis.

Neck surgery is extremely dangerous and seldom successful. Increased pain and/or quadriplegia have resulted too many times from surgery undertaken to relieve residual symptoms of whiplash.

To maximize the benefits of acupuncture and prevent the development of arthritis, patients should take at least two grams of Vitamin C and 200 mg. of Pantothenic acid daily. They should avoid vitamin capsules and tablets which contain iron or copper.

Acupuncture points for relieving whiplash residuals include:

Meridian points: Lu 7 · Co 11, 15, and 16 · SI 3 and 19 · GB 39 · UB 10, 60, and 62 · GB 20 and 39

Auricular points: Neck · Shoulder · Sympathy · Lung

DISC PROBLEMS AND SPINAL ABNORMALITIES

The intervertebral discs, especially between the fourth and fifth lumbar vertebrae, are subject to stress which leads to degenerative changes. Symptoms of back pain arise when surrounding vertebral ligaments are damaged or displaced, allowing disc material to protrude and cause nerve root irritation and pressure. In most cases, rupture or herniation of an intervertebral disc is caused by injury. Lifting with the trunk in a flexed position, or exertion with the back in an unusual alignment or posture, are recognized as precipitating factors. The resulting defect may become apparent immediately or be delayed for months or years.

Congenital abnormalities of the spine, or acquired abnormalities from polio, injuries, or surgery, predispose to disc problems. People with spina bifida, scoliosis, and kyphosis are likely to have episodes of pain from disc pathology causing nerve and muscle irritation. Acupuncture cannot correct these abnormalities, but it can relieve the pain and improve the general physiology of the structures involved to make the episodes of pain less frequent and discourage the development of arthritis.

The most common sites for intervertebral disc rupture are in the lumbosacral region. Herniation occasionally occurs in the cervical spine and very rarely in the thoracic region. The symptoms and signs associated with a degenerated or ruptured intervertebral disc depend on the location and size of the herniation.

It is important to rule out spinal tumors, which should be removed promptly, before acupuncture is attempted. If a spinal tumor is present, acupuncture will not relieve the symptoms.

The acupuncture treatment of disc pathology is similar to that for arthritis and myopathy causing similar symptoms. Before subjecting a patient to the hazards of laminectomy or even a myelogram for disc pathology, acupuncture should be given a chance to relieve the symptoms. It may relieve muscle spasms which are aggravating the condition. It should be remembered that a person may function well and be pain-free despite disc pathology. Acupuncture is safer than many diagnostic procedures, including myelograms. It is also safer than traction and bed rest since such inactivity may result in thrombosis of leg veins.

Surgical intervention is seldom necessary for degenerative disc disease. Subsequent spinal fusion is often performed about two years after disc surgery if the patient attempts to lift anything heavy or engages in strenuous exercise. Many of these operations are unsuccessful and leave the patient with worse pain and disability. Some patients have five or more laminectomies, each time desperately hoping that the next surgical procedure will bring relief but actually having more residual pain and disability after each operation.

Before attempting surgery, a physician should remind himself that all surgery destroys tissue and may lead to infection, other undesirable side effects, a period of pain, discomfort, and disability for his patient. He should also remember that all chemical anesthetics are poisonous and potentially lethal.

Most symptoms of lumbar disc pathology can be relieved by six to ten acupuncture treatments. The acupuncture points can be used bilaterally and potentiated with 50–150 microamperes of pulsating current. The standard acupuncture points can be combined with points for depression or other problems as indicated. Usually 12–16 needles should be inserted for each treatment.

The standard points are:

For cervical problems

Meridian points:	Co 4 · SI 12–15 · UB 10–12 · Br 12 · St 13, 14, and 36 · Sp 6
Auricular points:	Neck · Shenmen · Sympathy · Shoulder

For thoracic problems

Meridian points:	Co 4, 14, 15, and 16 · SI 14 and 15 · GB 25 · UB 12–22, and 36–47 · Br 4–11
Auricular points:	Thoracic · Lumbar · Shenmen

For lumbar problems

Meridian points:	Co 4 · St 36 · Br 3–5 · UB 20–28, 31, 47, and 48 · GB 30
Auricular points:	Lumbar · Shenmen · Sacral · Coccygeal

BACKACHE

Almost everybody suffers from backache occasionally because it can result from normal activities. The most frequent cause of backache is muscle strain from hard work or strenuous exercise. Usually this type of backache is relieved by a few days of decreased activity. Backaches which are extremely painful or last more than a few days require thorough diagnostic studies to determine whether they are caused by a condition which might require prompt medical or surgical treatment, such as tumors, fractures, kidney, or gall bladder disease. Tumors of the spinal cord may cause severe backache but are often benign, and it is important to diagnose and remove them surgically as early as possible. Acupuncture will not give lasting relief from backaches caused by such conditions.

Spinal disc pathology—slipped or degenerative discs—may produce severe pain in the neck or lumbar area and radiate down the arms or legs. Cervical disc pathology is often caused by "whiplash" injuries in automobile accidents. Pain from a slipped lumbar disc may come on suddenly when a person bends over and then hurts too much to straighten up again immediately. Bed rest with traction is considered conservative treatment for slipped or degenerative discs, but it is often unsuccessful and may lead to thrombosis of the leg veins. Surgery for slipped and degenerative discs is hazardous and sometimes makes the backache more severe. Even if disc surgery relieves the pain, the relief may last only two years and then have to be followed by a spinal fusion. This is likely to produce malalignment of other parts of the spine and result in more slipped discs. Surgery on the spine also encourages the development of osteoarthritis there, which increases pain and disability.

Some patients have had as many as ten back operations before coming to the Washington Acupuncture Center for relief of backaches. They explain that each time before surgery they were persuaded that one more operation would relieve their pain. Many patients found temporary relief of back pain by taking increasing doses of narcotics and became addicted to them. The narcotics spoiled their appetites and made them too depressed to eat properly. Malnutrition, therefore, frequently accompanies backaches and taking drugs for pain relief. On the other hand, some people eat and drink excessively in an attempt to compensate for their pain and related depression. Obesity puts an added strain on the back and increases pain. Patients with backache should be treated with appropriate diet and vitamin therapy along with acupuncture.

Any injury to the back from automobile accidents, falls, or other trauma may result in osteoarthritis of the spine with pinching of spinal nerves. Surgery for this condition may give temporary relief but will lead to more arthritis with increased pain later. Any of the drugs which relieve the symptoms of osteoarthritis may have dangerous and even fatal side effects.

Rheumatoid arthritis of the spine, spondylitis or Marie-Strümpell disease may begin spontaneously, especially in young men, and can be crippling as well as painful. It is generally aggravated by surgery but may be considerably relieved by acupuncture. Cortisone or its derivatives may relieve the arthritis symptoms but create a drug dependence more dangerous than narcotic dependence. Corticoid drugs suppress the patient's adrenal glands, and a fatal adrenal crisis may result if they are discontinued abruptly. Corticoids also cause fluid retention and predispose people to diabetes. Most of the drugs which relieve the pain and stiffness of arthritis have undesirable side effects. Phenylbutazone (Butazolidin) can cause fatal aplastic anemia. Even aspirin causes stomach ulcers.

Various congenital defects of the spine may require surgical correction if severe, but acupuncture can often relieve the pain associated with minor congenital malformations. The body can adapt to considerable bony deformity without pain or significant disability.

Osteoporosis is decalcification of the bones including the spinal vertebrae and is usually found in people past 40. This condition may cause compression fractures of vertebrae with a loss of height and pain from pressure on the spinal nerves. It has been treated with sex hormones without much success in proportion to the undesirable side effects of such therapy. Megavitamin and appropriate mineral therapy may be more effective and is unlikely to produce undesirable side effects. Acupuncture can relieve the pain from this condition and can be given along with nutritional therapy.

Multiple myeloma is a malignant plasmocytoma which should be diagnosed and given appropriate anticancer treatment as promptly as possible. It causes destruction of the vertebrae and severe pain. Cancer of any part of the body can metastasize to the spine and cause severe pain. Acupuncture should not be used to treat any type of cancer or malignancy. However, it can be used in place of narcotics to relieve severe pain while other appropriate treatment is being given, but it may have to be repeated once or twice a day to relieve the pain of terminal cancer.

The acupuncture treatment of backaches usually includes the following standard points regardless of the cause of the backache, but the skilled acupuncturist will add other points or omit some of these depending on the location and cause of the pain and his evaluation of the patient as a whole before each treatment. Lasting relief of pain from muscle strain or sprain, disc pathology, scoliosis, kyphosis, spina bifida, or any type of arthritis is usually obtained by the time six to ten treatments have been given. Many patients experience relief from pain during their first treatment by a highly skilled acupuncturist. More acupuncture treatments may be required to control pain from malignancies or other progressive disorders.

The needles are usually inserted bilaterally and may be potentiated by 50–200 microamperes of sawtooth or square wave pattern electricity. The standard points for backache are:

Meridian points: UB 10–48 · Br 3–14 · SI 14 and 15 · GB 30, 34, and 39 · Ki 1 and 3

Auricular points: Thoracic · Lumbar · Sacral · Coccygeal · Kidney · Shenmen · Sympathy

TENDINITIS AND TENOSYNOVITIS

Tendinitis is inflammation of a tendon. Tenosynovitis is inflammation of the sheath of a tendon, which contains lubricating fluid. Both conditions are frequently found together in rheumatic diseases or may result from muscle and joint injuries, systemic or local infections, or metabolic disorders. The most common problem areas are the shoulder, wrist, hip, knee, and heel (achilles tendon).

Injection of cortisone derivatives and procaine may relieve symptoms but can result in nerve irritation and can aggravate the symptoms. Sometimes surgery is performed for what is considered to be "stenosing tenosynovitis," but this may make symptoms worse. Application of heat or cold is not usually helpful, and splinting may lead to calcification and reduced mobility. Drugs are ineffective, except for temporary analgesia, and may have undesirable side effects.

Acupuncture usually relieves pain and stiffness after the first few treatments. It cannot remove calcium deposits, but it can improve metabolism in conjunction with nutritional therapy, which should be continued after acupuncture is completed. Six to ten acupuncture treatments are usually adequate for lasting relief. Nutritional therapy should include Vitamins C, D, and E, Pantothenate, and Biotin. Specific doses should be prescribed by physicians.

Selection of acupuncture points for treating tendinitis and tenosynovitis depend somewhat on the location of the tendons involved. Points should be selected to relieve pain in the involved area along with Co 5 · Lu 7 · Va 7 · He 7 for arm and hand muscles; GB 30 for hip muscles; GB 34 for knee tendons; and GB 39 for ankle tendons. (See the table on "Specific Points for Various Conditions.")

TENNIS ELBOW

Tennis elbow is radiohumeral bursitis or epicondylitis caused by muscle strain in such motions as hitting a tennis ball or using a screwdriver. It may be extremely painful and disable the arm involved. Weakness of the wrist in dorsiflexion may accompany the elbow pain.

X-ray findings may be negative but sometimes reveal periostitis. Injections of procaine or hydrocortisone into the most painful area may give temporary relief but may increase the pain in some cases. Surgical intervention may result in permanent disability and is unlikely to be successful. Immobilizing the arm in a splint may relieve the pain but result in persistent limitation of elbow mobility and muscle atrophy. Analgesic medications strong enough to relieve the pain may have dangerous side effects and may be habit forming.

Acupuncture is a safe and effective treatment for tennis elbow. Six treatments are usually enough for lasting relief. Until the treatments are completed, it is advisable not to play tennis or use the involved arm for other strenuous exercise or heavy lifting. Some athletes, however, have had enough relief from the first few treatments to be able to resume their regular schedules. Points for treating tennis elbow include:

Meridian points: Co 5, 11, and 12 · Lu 7 · Va 7 · He 7 · GB 34

Auricular points: Elbow · Shenmen · Sympathy

Increasing the protein content of the diet and supplementing it with vitamins and minerals may improve muscle, bone, and joint physiology.

MUSCLE STRAINS AND SPASMS

Muscle pain from strains, sprains, or spasms may be disabling. Using a muscle to lift something in an awkward position may tear muscle fibers with bleeding into muscle tissue and injury to nerves there. This type of muscle injury is usually referred to as a strain. Severe muscle strain involving tendons and sometimes the tearing of ligaments around a joint is called a sprain.

Muscle spasms may be produced by nerve irritation from muscle strains and sprains and by neurologic disorders not related to injuries. They may follow strokes or spinal injuries and are a serious problem for many hemiplegics and paraplegics.

Whatever the cause of muscle strains or spasms, acupuncture is a safe and effective treatment for relieving them. Some patients experience considerable relief after the first treatment, but many more treatments may be required for lasting relief. Six treatments are usually enough to relieve pain from muscle strain permanently.

Nutritional deficiencies may produce or aggravate muscle spasms. To facilitate recovery, patients should take the following daily during and after acupuncture. Vitamins B1 (30 mg.), B2 (30 mg.), B6 (30 mg.), C (2 gm.), D (400 units), E (400 units), and calcium (2 gm.) along with a diet high in protein and low in carbohydrates and fat. Other vitamin and mineral supplements prescribed by a physician may also be beneficial.

Strenuous exercise and chilling should be avoided, but mild exercise and heat may be beneficial in moderation.

Acupuncture point selection depends on the location of symptoms. Points for relief of pain in the area involved should be included. Points for relieving muscle strains and spasms in some areas include the following:

Neck

Meridian points: SI 3 · UB 10, 60, and 62 · GB 20 and 37

Auricular points: Neck · Shoulder · Shenmen

Shoulder

Meridian points: Co 14–16 · SI 3, 11, 12, and 19 · GB 21

Auricular points: Shoulder · Neck · Shenmen

Arms and Hands

Meridian points: Lu 9 and 10 · Va 8 · Co 3 and 4 · Me 2–4 · GB 21

Auricular points: Fingers · Shoulder · Elbow · Neck · Sympathy

Thoracic and Lumbar

Meridian points: SI 14 and 15 · UB 12–24 and 37–47 · St 36 · Sp 6

Auricular points: Thoracic · Lumbar · Shenmen

BURSITIS

Bursitis is inflammation of a bursa, which is a fibrous sac containing fluid located around a joint and acting as a cushion. Bursae are located where tendons pass over bony prominences. Bursitis may result from injury, malnutrition or diseases, such as arthritis. The walls of the bursae may calcify from chronic irritation and not heal properly, especially if a person has a deficiency of Vitamins C, D, and Pantothenic acid.

This condition is painful and limits the movement of the joint involved. The shoulder, elbow, heel, and knee joints are the ones most commonly involved. Some surgeons will attempt to cut away the calcium, but it usually returns as a response to the surgical injury.

Injecting hydrocortisone directly into the bursa is usually painful, but it will reduce the inflammation temporarily. The pain may be relieved for as long as a month by this procedure if it is performed skillfully, but in many cases, attempts at such injections aggravate the symptoms.

Acupuncture is usually effective for relieving pain and stiffness from bursitis. Six treatments are enough in most cases. Taking the vitamins mentioned above, drinking plenty of water, avoiding coffee, tea, cola, alcohol, and chilling will improve metabolism and discourage calcification of the bursae. Points for treating bursitis include:

Shoulder

      Meridian points: Co 11, 15, and 16 · SI 19 · UB 39

      Auricular points: Shoulder · Shenmen

Elbow

      Meridian points: Co 11 · St 36 · GB 21

      Auricular points: Elbow · Shenmen

Knee

      Meridian points: St 34 and 35 · St 41 · UB 54 · GB 39, 40, and 54 · Li 4 and 8

      Auricular points: Knee · Shenmen · Sympathy

Ischial Tuberosity

      Meridian points: GB 30 · UB 30, 33, 34, 35, 48, 49, and 50

      Auricular points: Hip · Lumbar · Sacral

Heel

      Meridian points: UB 60, 61, and 62 · Ki 3–6 · Li 4 · Sp 5 and 6 · St 36 and 41

      Auricular points: Ankle · Toes · Sacral

chapter 20

NEUROLOGIC DISORDERS

Acupuncture is effective for treating some neurologic disorders that many neurology textbooks label as hopeless without chance of remission. It may also relieve pain from many diseases, including cancer and various types of neuralgia and neuritis.

Treatment of pain from arthritis and related diseases is discussed under the section on musculo-skeletal disorders. In a sense, all pain is neurologic, but relief of pain from various causes is discussed in other sections as well.

Although many neurologic disorders give symptoms of impaired function as well as pain, neurologic disorders are classified here according to which set of symptoms is usually predominant. No classification of neurologic disorders is entirely satisfactory. To determine which points to use for treating a specific patient, several different articles might be referred to.

IMPAIRED FUNCTION SYNDROMES

The ability of acupuncture to improve the function of impaired parts of the body is less well understood than its ability to relieve pain. The results of improved function, however, are much more demonstrable and usually measurable.

Improving the function of a part of the body usually takes many more acupuncture treatments than relieving pain does. In cases where there is a dramatic return of a body function after only one acupuncture treatment, a hysterical etiology should be suspected. In most cases, return of function is slow and requires ten or more treatments for significant improvement.

Acupuncture will not restore severed nerves or a completely transected spinal cord. In many cases, however, it is not known whether nerve tissue has been completely destroyed or merely damaged. In such cases, a trial of ten acupuncture treatments should produce some significant improvement in function if there is a possibility that function can be restored. In China, however, acupuncturists may not give up treating a person for paralysis until they have given him at least 100 acupuncture treatments.

Attempts at classifying impaired function syndromes are difficult because some involve intellectual, sensory, and motor function. In some cases of brain damage, such as cerebral palsy, intellectual function may be better than average. For this reason, cerebral palsy is classified as impaired motor function. Many people with seizures or hypersomnia also function unusually well intellectually, but people with these disorders usually do not have impaired motor or sensory function. Hypersomnia and seizures are therefore classified under Organic Brain Syndromes because their symptoms are thought to be caused by brain pathology.

Organic Brain Syndromes

Deficiencies of memory, cognition, orientation, attention span, judgment, or affect caused by organic brain pathology may respond to acupuncture combined with psychotherapy and nutritional therapy. Many elderly and middle-aged people become depressed about the loss of loved ones, loneliness, unemployment, and physical ailments which cause pain and disability. Antidepressant drugs and tranquilizers usually aggravate their symptoms. Narcotics prescribed to relieve their pain and self-medication with alcohol make them feel better temporarily but increase their dementia. They lose interest in food and other things they used to enjoy because they feel unloved, unwanted, unsuccessful, hopeless, and helpless. Their body energy is progressively diminished as *Yin* exceeds *Yang*. It is important to treat their physical ailments along with trying to improve their mental state.

Acupuncture should be directed at restoring their balance of body energy by stimulation to increase *Yang* and reduce *Yin*. Some patients may respond dramatically to the first few treatments if they don't have serious problems of drug withdrawal, malnutrition, or somatic diseases. Others may require as many as 30 acupuncture treatments for optimal benefit. Points to use include:

Meridian points: St 25 and 36 · He 7 · UB 15, 18, and 20 · Br 4, 14, and 20 · Ki 4 · Sx 2, 5, 14, and 23 · Sp 3, 6, and 15 · Me 6

Auricular points: Brain · Lung · Liver · Kidney · Spleen · Heart · Gonads

AMNESIA

Both psychogenic and neurogenic amnesia have been treated effectively with acupuncture. Patients with hysterical amnesia often respond dramatically after one treatment, while people whose amnesia results from head trauma or strokes will respond more slowly and are much less likely to have their memories restored completely.

Acupuncture, of course, should not be used to treat amnesia in a person with a recent head injury until appropriate diagnostic studies, including skull X-rays, electroencephalogram, and brain scan, have been performed. People who have amnesia from strokes or surgical procedures will usually not seek treatment for amnesia until its etiology is well established. Psychotherapy or environmental stimulation and nutritional therapy should be given along with acupuncture to help restore the patient's memory. Electropotentiation is usually beneficial but not essential.

The acupuncture points for amnesia treatment are:

Meridian points: St 36 · He 7 · UB 15 · Co 4 · Br 20

Auricular points: Brain · Lung · Liver · Kidney · Spleen · Heart · Gonads

APHASIA

Aphasia is a speech disorder usually caused by brain pathology. Various types of aphasia may result from strokes, trauma, or surgery with damage to the brain, but aphasia can also be psychogenic. Both psychologic and neurologic aphasia are usually accompanied by some degree of amnesia. For this reason, it is advisable to use the acupuncture points for amnesia along with those for aphasia. Psychotherapy and speech therapy are also important in restoring the patient's ability to speak.

The acupuncture points for aphasia are:

Meridian points: Co 4 · St 6 · Sx 14 and 23

Auricular points: same as for Organic Brain Syndrome

Points for treating anxiety, depression, and other symptoms can be used along with these. Electropotentiation may be helpful but is not essential. A course of six to ten treatments usually results in significant improvement but may have to be repeated monthly until speech approaches normal.

DEMENTIA

Dementia is loss of intellectual faculties, reasoning power, memory, and will due to degeneration of brain tissue. It is characterized by confusion, disorientation, confabulation, apathy, and stupor of varying degrees. It is often associated with old age but may develop earlier in life.

Presenile dementia may be diagnosed as Alzheimer's disease, brain atrophy demonstrable by pneumoencephalogram, or axial tomography of the brain. People with high intelligence who have held positions of great respect and responsibility may become afflicted with this disorder and cause serious problems. A physician or judge who develops Alzheimer's disease may make disastrous mistakes before he is forced to retire. No drug or surgical treatment is considered effective.

Acupuncture, along with nutritional therapy, can improve brain physiology and thereby relieve some of the symptoms of dementia. Most patients treated for dementia at the Washington Acupuncture Center have shown significant improvement in mental status. Many of them have been treated for other medical problems at the same time. Some of them begin to function rationally after the first few treatments, but others require many more treatments for maximum benefit.

Drugs given to control behavior may cause further brain damage, ataxia, dyskinesia, and convulsions. They usually do much more harm than good and should be discontinued as soon as possible without causing withdrawal symptoms.

Since dementia is often preceded by hypoglycemia and cerebral arteriosclerosis, a high protein diet low in fat and carbohydrates should be given.

Vitamins and minerals especially important in treating dementia include: A (10,000 International Units), B1 (50 mg.), B2 (50 mg.), B6 (50 mg.), B12 (100 mcg.), Biotin (20 mcg.), Choline (50 mg.), Folic acid (0.4 mg.), Inositol (50 mg.), Niacinamide (1000 mg.), Pangamic acid (50 mg.), Pantothenic acid (100 mg.), C (2 gm.), D (800 International Units), E (400 International Units), Calcium (200 mg.), Magnesium (200 mg.), Selenium (20 mcg.), and Zinc (20 mg.) daily. Many of these nutrients may be combined in single capsules or tablets but are not adequately available in food at the present time. Food processing and additives have made it necessary to take vitamin and mineral capsules or tablets daily for optimal nutrition.

Acupuncture points for dementia include:

Meridian points: Co 4 · St 6 and 36 · He 7 · UB 15 · Br 14 and 20

Auricular points: same as for Organic Brain Syndrome

COMA

Coma is unconsciousness from which a person cannot be aroused by ordinary methods. It may be due to intracranial disorders, such as trauma, drugs, toxins, hypoxia, metabolic deficiencies, circulatory, respiratory, or temperature disturbances. In cases of severe brain damage, acupuncture is not effective.

After careful diagnosis, all standard American treatments should be performed before acupuncture is attempted.

The acupuncture points used for arousing people from coma include:

Meridian points: Br 20 and 26 · Sx 4 and 8 · Va 3, 6, and 9 · UB 15, 17, and 54 ·· He 7 and 9 · Li 3 · GB 30, 31, and 39 · Co 1, 4, and 11

Auricular points: Brain · Forehead · Shenmen · Sympathy Spleen · Kidney · Rectum

HYPERSOMNIA

Sleep disorders include sleeping too much (hypersomnia), sleeping at inappropriate times (catalepsy and narcolepsy), disturbed sleep patterns, and insomnia. Some people fall asleep when they laugh or after eating regardless of how important it may be for them to keep awake at such times. Others sleep a normal amount of time (4–8 hours) per night, but have periods of prolonged apnea during sleep or make kicking or convulsive movements while remaining asleep. Talking while asleep may be embarrassing but is less serious than walking while asleep, which may lead to falls and injuries. Some physicians consider sleepwalking and convulsive movements during sleep as epileptic equivalents, which should be treated with anti-epileptic drugs, as well as the acupuncture points for seizures.

Nightmares which do not lead to sleepwalking are generally considered normal. Almost everyone has unpleasant dreams occasionally. Repetition of the same disturbing dream many times may be an indication of serious emotional problems which should be treated with psychotherapy . Snoring is normal but may be relieved by acupuncture. The points for this are listed under "Insomnia."

Points for hypersomnia, catalepsy, and narcolepsy include:

Meridian points: Br 26 · Sx 4 and 8 · He 7 · UB 15 · Va 6 and 9 · Li 3

Auricular points: Brain · Forehead · Spleen · Stomach · Liver · Kidney · Shenmen

SEIZURES

Any type of convulsive episode involving all or part of the body is called a seizure. Even petit mal epilepsy—losses of consciousness lasting only a few seconds—may be considered a type of seizure although there are no convulsions with this disorder. Grand mal epilepsy is characterized by convulsions of the entire body with loss of consciousness. Epileptic equivalents are periods of deviant behavior during which the subject appears to be conscious but afterwards has no memory of his activities. Psychomotor seizures usually involve only parts of the body, sometimes without loss of consciousness.

Since Dilantin, Mysoline, Tridione, Phenobarbital, and various other drugs are usually effective in controlling seizures, acupuncture is only used to help control the seizures of patients for whom the drugs are inadequate. It may also be used to reduce the quantity of drugs patients have to take if they are having serious problems with side effects of these drugs. A patient should not stop taking his antiseizure drugs when he begins acupuncture treatments. He should only reduce them gradually on the advice of his physician.

Several series of ten to twelve treatments each are usually required for the acupuncture treatment of seizures. The points used include:

Meridian points: Gb 2, 13, 20, and 40 · Me 3, 5, and 17 · Co 4 and 10 · SI 3 and 19 · Li 2 · St 40 and 42 · Br 26 · UB 15, 18, and 62 · Sx 12 · Sp 6

Auricular points: Brain · Liver · Kidney · Shenmen · Sympathy

Impaired Sensory Perception

Impaired sensory perception usually detracts considerably from a person's ability to participate in vocational and recreational activities. He misses cues from his environment which warn him of danger or enable him to be appropriately responsive to pleasant stimulation.

Some sensory deficiencies are congenital while others are acquired as the result of injury or disease. In general, acupuncture is more likely to be effective for acquired sensory deficiencies but may be effective in some cases of congenital deficiencies.

By the time a person has had ten treatments for sensory deficiency, there should be some sign of improvement if acupuncture is going to be helpful. Optimal improvement may require many more treatments. Point selection for treating sensory deficiencies depends on the sense organs involved and the general health of the patient.

ANOSMIA

Anosmia, absence of the sense of smell, usually results from damage to the olfactory nerves, which lie under the frontal lobes of the brain. This may be caused by a space-occupying mass in the brain and should, therefore, be investigated by such diagnostic studies as Computerized Axial Tomography brain scan before acupuncture is attempted. Brain tumors or hematomas require prompt surgical removal. Tumors of the nasopharyngeal region may also cause anosmia and should be removed as soon as possible. Any abnormality of the sense of smell should be regarded as a possible warning of a life-threatening neurosurgical problem. Many causes of anosmia, however, do not require surgical intervention and can be safely treated by acupuncture.

Dietary zinc deficiency may diminish the sense of smell, and it is, therefore, important to prescribe this mineral along with other essential minerals and vitamins while treating anosmia with acupuncture. Psychological causes of anosmia should also be considered and treated by psychotherapy as indicated. Acupuncture points for treating anxiety and nasal allergies should be used for at least some of the treatments.

The most frequently used points for treating anosmia are:

Meridian points: Co 4 and 20 · Br 14, 16, 23, and 26 · SI 2 · UB 13

Auricular points: Brain · Kidney · Eye · Internal Nose

Although some cases may respond after the first few treatments, 30 or more treatments may be required.

NEUROGENIC BLINDNESS

If the eyeball is still intact, acupuncture may relieve neurogenic blindness. Diagnosis and prompt appropriate treatment are especially important with eye problems, however, and acupuncture should not be the treatment of first choice for most intraeyeball problems.

Glaucoma (increased intraocular pressure) is a frequent cause of blindness which can usually be controlled by early treatment with drugs or surgery. Cataracts (opaque lenses) can be removed surgically. There is some evidence, however, that acupuncture can improve eye physiology and has even been helpful in treating glaucoma and cataracts. It can be used in conjunction with chemical treatment of glaucoma and to discourage the development of incipient cataracts.

Points for treating glaucoma and cataracts are:

Meridian points: GB 4, 5, 6, and 14 · St 2 · UB 2, and 3 · Me 4 · Li 4 · Sx 24

Auricular points: Eye · Eye I · Eye II · Liver · Kidney

Retinitis pigmentosa is a progressive deterioration of the retina, for which there is no effective standard medical or surgical treatment. Acupuncture may be helpful in some cases of this disease. The points listed above are used.

Blindness from optic nerve pathology, nerve damage from prenatal rubella, birth trauma, or postnatal diseases may respond well to acupuncture.

Brain tumors putting pressure on the optic nerve should, of course, be ruled out by appropriate diagnostic tests before acupuncture is attempted. After removal of a brain tumor, however, the optic nerve may have residual damage and not function adequately until after acupuncture treatment.

Lesions of the optic nerve or of the nerves controlling the eye muscles from multiple sclerosis usually respond well to acupuncture. Diplopia (double vision) may be relieved after only two or three treatments.

Classical acupuncture points used for improving the function of these nerves include:

Meridian points: Lu 10 · Co 14 · SI 17 and 18 · Li 3 · Br 20 and
                   24

Auricular points: Eye · Eye I · Eye II

Acupuncture needles are, of course, not inserted into the eyes. Some of the points used are on the arms or legs. Many patients have their vision restored by the time they have had six treatments, but others require many more for maximum benefit.

NEUROGENIC DEAFNESS

Neurogenic deafness is hearing deficiency resulting from damage to the auditory nervous system from the nerve fibers at the base of the cochlear hair cells up to and including the brain stem. This nerve damage may occur before birth or at any time during a person's life. It may affect just one side or both sides.

Until the effectiveness of acupuncture was demonstrated in the United States, doctors here thought that there was no effective treatment for nerve deafness. Hearing aids can make sounds louder but not more meaningful. For this reason, many people with nerve deafness don't use them. They amplify all sounds equally and may make the discrimination of words more difficult as well as subjecting the wearer to loud, unpleasant noises conducive to anxiety. By improving a person's ability to discriminate between different sounds and words, acupuncture can enable him to use a hearing aid more effectively even if the decibel level of sounds he hears does not improve.

Records of patients treated at the Washington Acupuncture Center in 1973 and 1974 indicated that over 90% of those with some residual hearing showed some improvement in discrimination. Over 70% showed at least a 10-decibel improvement at four or more frequencies as well on audiograms taken after ten treatments. Half of the patients who did not show improvement after the first ten treatments showed improvement in both discrimination and decibel level at some frequencies by the twentieth treatment.

Most patients receiving acupuncture for nerve deafness have one treatment a day. Some people between the ages of 12 and 50 are able to have two treatments a day. Others only receive treatments once or twice a week. The patients who receive treatments more frequently tend to get somewhat better results, but many people who have only had treatments once a week have shown significant improvement by their tenth treatment. Occasionally a patient will experience a dramatic return to normal hearing after less than five treatments, some even after the first treatment. Most people, however, require at least ten treatments to show significant improvement and many more treatments to obtain optimal improvement.

The patients most likely to show rapid improvement in hearing with acupuncture treatments are older people who have lost their hearing gradually. Some teenagers hear much better after only a few treatments, but young children usually improve more slowly, often requiring forty or more treatments for optimal results. We have successfully treated nerve deafness caused by many different factors, including prenatal rubella, RH incompatibility, meningitis, viral infections, loud noises, and presbycusis.

Acupuncture points for treating deafness include:

Meridian points: Co 4 · SI 19 · UB 23 · Me 3, 5, 17, and 22 · GB 11 and 12

TINNITUS

Endogenous noises which a person hears—ringing, hissing, or roaring in his head—are called tinnitus. This condition may accompany loss of hearing and be constant or intermittent. An attempt to determine the cause of tinnitus is very important because many of its causes respond to antibiotics or other standard American treatments. Drugs, such as quinine, streptomycin, salicylates, and alcohol may cause tinnitus. These should be eliminated before acupuncture is started. Many cases are caused by illness from which the patient has otherwise recovered.

Acupuncture has a high rate of effectiveness in the relief of tinnitus. Usually the condition is relieved by the time ten treatments have been given, and the relief may last for years. Vitamin E (400 International Units), Vitamin B12 (200 mcg.), Niacinamide (500 mg.) and Vitamin C (2000 mg.) should be prescribed for the patient to take each day indefinitely, along with a low fat, low carbohydrate diet and other nutrients as indicated.

The acupuncture points for treating tinnitus are:

Meridian points: Co 4 and 5 · SI 4 and 5 · UB 23 · Ki 6 · Va 9 · Me 17 · GB 11 and 12

MENIERE'S DISEASE

Meniere's disease, a disorder of the inner ear, is characterized by episodes of deafness, tinnitus, vertigo, ataxia, nausea, and vomiting. The patient tends to fall toward the involved ear and becomes depressed about his disability.

Antibiotics should be given to clear up any ear infection. Drugs, such as atropine, scopolamine, dimenhydrinate, or antihistamines may be helpful but have undesirable side effects. While the disease usually responds somewhat to antibiotics, the episodes of dizziness are very resistant to medical treatment.

Surgery or ultrasound to destroy the labyrinth relieves the vertigo and nausea but increases deafness. Such hazardous procedures may also cause brain and facial nerve damage. It is important that this disease be differentiated from acoustic neuroma, which requires surgical treatment for tumor removal before acupuncture is used to treat residual symptoms. If the patient's symptoms are due to a tumor, surgery is indicated. Correct diagnosis is, therefore, especially important.

Acupuncture is a safe and effective treatment for Meniere's disease after any infection has been cleared up with antibiotics. Six to ten treatments will give lasting relief in most cases. Since Meniere's disease tends to be recurrent, however, another series of acupuncture treatments may be required years or months later.

Nutritional therapy including Niacinamide, Lecithin, and Vitamins A, C, and E should be started along with acupuncture. Individual requirements can be prescribed by acupuncture center physicians.

Acupuncture points for treating Meniere's disease include:

Meridian points: Co 4 and 5 · SI 4 and 5 · UB 23 · Ki 6 · Va 9 · Me 17 · GB 11 and 12

Auricular points: Inner Ear · Brain · Shenmen

DIZZINESS

Dizziness is a term often used to describe ataxia, vertigo, or difficulty in maintaining balance. It is an unpleasant sensation of disturbed relations with surrounding objects in space. *Ataxia* is impaired coordination of voluntary muscular action, especially the groups of muscles used for walking or reaching for objects with the hands. It is caused by pathology of central or peripheral nervous system pathways involved in balancing muscle movements. *Vertigo* is the sensation that one's nearby environment is revolving around him or that he is revolving around it.

Alcohol or other drugs can cause temporary dizziness, ataxia, and vertigo, but if these symptoms persist for more than 24 hours after the last dose of the drug, thorough diagnostic studies are required.

Prolonged alcoholism can cause persistent ataxia with cerebellar degeneration, which may be somewhat relieved by megavitamin therapy and acupuncture. Tranquilizers, such as Thorazine, Mellaril, or Haldol, may damage the basal ganglia of the brain, thereby causing persistent ataxia.

Acupuncture can be used to treat alcoholism and as an effective substitute for psychotropic drugs in treating mental illness. It can also relieve the ataxia and dyskinesia caused by these drugs.

Multiple sclerosis is a frequent cause of ataxia with or without a sensation of dizziness. Although cortisone and some other drugs may give some temporary relief of multiple sclerosis symptoms, they have serious side effects and do more harm than good if taken over a long period of time. Acupuncture is the safest and most effective treatment for multiple sclerosis.

Symptoms of dizziness, ataxia, and vertigo are usually relieved by the time six to ten acupuncture treatments have been given. For progressive neurological disorders such as multiple sclerosis, however, a series of treatments every few months may be required for continued remission of symptoms.

Classical points on the front of the body include:

Meridian points: Br 24 · GB 14 and 24 · Li 14 · He 2 · Lu 6 · Sp 12, 36, 40, 41, and 44

Points on the back of the body include:

Meridian points: UB 8 · GB 9 and 21 · Br 14, 17, and 19 · Me 11 · Co 14 · Ki 6 and 10

NUMBNESS

Numbness is absence of feeling. It can be produced temporarily by chemical anesthetics. Persistent lack of feeling in any part of the body, however, indicates a neurologic disorder.

Severing any nerve with a sensory component will result in numbness peripherally. Acupuncture cannot repair severed nerves. Many cases of numbness, however, result from non-severing injury or pressure on a nerve. Acupuncture can be very effective for treating such conditions, especially after spinal injuries.

Restoring feeling and function takes many more acupuncture treatments than relieving pain. A few patients experience a dramatic return of feeling during the first treatment, and some experience this after six treatments. Others need more than 20 treatments before their numbness is relieved.

When numbness accompanies paralysis, return of feeling to the involved part often comes before return of function. The first sensation is usually one of warmth followed by a period of paresthesia, which may be somewhat uncomfortable until normal feeling is established.

Diagnostic procedures to determine the cause of numbness and appropriate treatment, if available, should be undertaken before acupuncture. Nutritional therapy may be helpful along with acupuncture. It can be prescribed by supervising physicians.

Acupuncture points for relieving numbness include:

Meridian points: St 36 · Sp 4 · Ki 1 · Br 25

Auricular points: Brain · Liver · Kidney

Upper extremities

Meridian point: Co 10, 11, and 15 · GB 21

Lower extremities

Meridian points: UB 23, 31, and 34 · GB 30, 31, 34, 36, and 39 · Ki 3 · Br 14

Impaired Motor Function

Impaired motor function is loss of the ability to move or to control the movement of various parts of the body. It includes all degrees of paralysis, deficiencies of muscular coordination, muscle spasms, loss of muscle strength, tremors and other involuntary movements.

Complete paralysis accompanied by complete loss of sensation in any part of the body may mean that the spinal cord, or major nerve leading to that part of the body, has been severed. Acupuncture cannot restore severed nerves. If the paralysis and sensation loss is not complete, however, there is a good chance that acupuncture may produce considerable improvement in function. Even in some cases of complete paralysis, acupuncture may restore function if the spinal cord or major nerve has only been damaged rather than severed.

Causes of impaired motor function include injuries to the brain or spinal cord from trauma, surgery, tumors, strokes, oxygen deprivation, bacterial invasion, and progressive neurologic or systemic diseases. It is important to identify the cause and arrange for any available appropriate treatment before, or at the same time as, acupuncture is given to relieve symptoms.

Restoration of motor function usually takes much longer than relieving pain or emotional disorders. Some patients may notice improvement of function during, or after, their first treatment. Most of them will notice some significant improvement by the time they have had ten treatments. But many more treatments are usually required for maximal improvement in motor function.

Diaphragm

> Meridian points: UB 17 · Li 14 · Sx 15
>
> Auricular points: Diaphragm · Lung · Thoracic

Abdominal muscles

> Meridian points: UB 20 and 21 · St 21 and 25
>
> Auricular points: Abdomen · Thoracic · Diaphragm · Lung · Hip

Upper extremities

> Meridian points: Ex 17 · Co 4, 6, and 11 · Me 5
>
> Auricular points: Shoulder · Elbow · Fingers · Neck

Lower extremities

> Meridian points: Ex 21 · GB 30 and 34 · UB 40 · Li 8 · St 36, 37, and 41 · Ki 3 · Sp 6
>
> Auricular points: Lumbar · Sacral · Hip · Knee · Ankle · Toes

Urethral and rectal sphincters

> Meridian points: Sx 4 · UB 32 and 54

AMYOTROPHIC LATERAL SCLEROSIS

Amyotrophic lateral sclerosis (ALS) is a neurologic disease which becomes evident in adult life, usually between the ages of 20 and 60. It is characterized by progressive muscle weakness and atrophy first noticed in the hands or the throat. The legs and muscles in all parts of the body eventually become involved, but the mind remains clear. This is the disease which afflicted famous baseball player Lou Gehrig and is therefore often referred to as "Lou Gehrig's Disease." Medical research has not yet discovered the cause or cure for this disease, which is being diagnosed at an increasing rate in the United States.

Although the average life expectancy after diagnosis of ALS is three years, the Washington Acupuncture Center has been treating some patients with ALS for more than four years with improvement rather than deterioration in their condition during this period. Most medical and neurology textbooks state that improvement never takes place with ALS, that there are no remissions, and that no medical treatment or physiotherapy techniques are effective.

Guanadine and snake venom have been considered effective in a few cases but have caused undesirable side effects and have not been accepted as good treatment by most neurologists. Some researchers have found Vitamin E, other vitamins, and various diets helpful. At least these are harmless and should improve general health. Megavitamin therapy can be given along with acupuncture.

Several courses of ten to twenty acupuncture treatments are required for this serious neurologic disorder. Patients who live nearby come for maintenance treatments on a weekly or monthly basis.

Before each treatment their condition is reevaluated to determine which acupuncture points should be used for that treatment. Electric potentiation of 30–50 microamperes is usually used with some of the needles. Needles are left in place 15–30 minutes. The points most frequently used are:

Meridian points: St 5, 10, and 11 · Li 16, 17, and 18 · Sx 22, 23, and 24 · Lu 2, 3, 6, and 10 · Sp 8, 9, 10, and 11 · Me 4, 9, 11, and 14 · SI 10, 12, and 15 · Co 3, 5, and 7

Auricular points: Pharynx · Larynx · Diaphragm · Elbow · Fingers · Neck · Thoracic · Lumbar · Liver · Lung

MULTIPLE SCLEROSIS

Multiple sclerosis is a slowly progressive neurologic disease with patches of demyelinization in the brain and spinal cord. Its cause is still uncertain, although the possibilities of viral etiology, autoimmune mechanisms, toxic agents, trauma, and hereditary metabolic factors have been considered. Its onset is insidious and usually occurs between the ages of 20 and 40. Because of the vagueness, transitory nature, and variety of early symptoms, the diagnosis may not be made until visual disturbances, ataxia, weakness of extremities, and difficulties with bladder control appear. Nystagmus, intention tremor, scanning speech, and euphoria are common symptoms. Expanding

cranial lesions, spinal cord tumors, syringomyelia, syphilis, and pernicious anemia should be ruled out before a patient is treated with
acupuncture.

Some of the drugs which have been prescribed for multiple sclerosis, such as cortisone derivatives, have caused serious adverse
reactions. Sometimes, however, they are dramatically effective for
treating acute exacerbations. Although improving a patient's general
health with vitamins may be helpful, there apparently is no other
treatment for multiple sclerosis as effective as acupuncture.

The acupuncture treatment of multiple sclerosis is aimed at
relieving its symptoms. Whether acupuncture can arrest the progress
of the disease is difficult to determine. It is impossible to explain scientifically at this time why acupuncture should be effective in multiple
sclerosis, but its rate of success in relieving symptoms is much higher
than could be expected from spontaneous remissions. Most patients
show significant improvement by the time they have had ten treatments. This improvement lasts for years in many cases but in others a
series of booster treatments as often as every 4–8 months is required
to maintain remission of symptoms. Patients are advised to return for
such treatments if an old symptom begins to recur or if a new one
develops.

The points for general treatment of multiple sclerosis are:

Meridian points: GB 20, 30, and 33 · UB 23, 54, and 60 · Sp 6
and 9 · Ki 3 · St 36 · Br 2

Other points are added for treatment of specific symptoms, such as
loss of bladder control or ataxia. The acupuncture points may be used
bilaterally and potentiated with 50–100 microamperes of pulsating
current. For each treatment 10–20 needles are inserted and left in
place for 20–30 minutes.

BELL'S PALSY

Bell's palsy is partial paralysis or paresis of the facial nerve. It is
usually characterized by difficulty in closing one eye and distortion of
the mouth toward the opposite side of the face. The cause is unknown,
but it is often associated with viral infections, exposure to cold, or
emotional stress.

Although this condition is not painful, it may make closing the eye
difficult and require a bandage or tape to protect the eye at night.
Sometimes it may be relieved within a week or month without treat-

ment other than rest, a nutritious diet, and vitamins. In many cases, however, the palsy persists for months or years and may involve both sides of the face.

Acupuncture will usually produce significant improvement by the time a patient has had six to ten treatments. These treatments should be taken daily or as close together as possible without more than a week between any two of them. The acupuncture points used will not be too close to the eye, and some of them may be on the arms or legs. During the course of treatment, the patient will begin to feel relaxed and free from tension and anxiety.

To obtain maximum benefit from acupuncture, the following vitamins are recommended during and following treatment: Vitamin B1 (50 mg), B2 (50 mg), B6 (50 mg), C (2 gm), D (400 International Units), and Calcium lactate (2 gm.) daily.

The classical acupuncture points used are:

Meridian points: SI 2, 4, 6, and 7 · Co 10, 11, 19, and 20 · St 18 and 36 · Br 16, 20, and 23 · UB 1 and 2 · GB 1, 3, 14, and 15 · Me 5, 15, 17, 22, and 23 · Sx 12 and 14 · Sp 6

Auricular points: Eye I and II · Maxillary Sinus · Brain · Liver · External Nose · Pharynx

It is of course not necessary or desirable to use all of these points for each treatment. Only 6–8 points should be used for the first treatment, and the others added later from time to time in accordance with the patient's response.

CEREBRAL PALSY

Cerebral palsy is a neurologic disorder caused by damage to the brain before, during, or soon after birth. Its comparatively high incidence in the United States may be related to the excessive use of obstetrical forceps and anesthetics which injure babies' brains.

Babies with cerebral palsy may appear normal during the first few weeks or months of life but often have difficulty nursing, vomit frequently, and are generally irritable. The diagnosis of cerebral palsy is usually made after the child has failed to sit up, crawl, or walk at the expected time. About 25% of cerebral palsy victims have convulsions, especially with febrile diseases, to which they are very susceptible.

Cases of cerebral palsy are divided into three types in accordance with the part of the brain which is thought to be most seriously damaged, but many have symptoms of more than one type. The "spastic" type have muscle spasms of their arms and legs which interfere with their walking or using their arms and hands effectively. Spasticity is associated with damage to the cerebral cortex. The "ataxic" type have difficulty maintaining their balance and are thought to have cerebellar damage. The "athetoid" type make purposeless involuntary movements which are indicative of damage to the basal ganglia. Although people with cerebral palsy have brain damage and may not speak, write, or perform manual tasks well, they may have high intelligence and are usually very sociable.

Drugs and surgery are generally ineffective in treating this disorder and may aggravate symptoms as well as producing other undesirable symptoms. Acupuncture is effective in reducing muscle spasms and improving coordination. Many children whose parents had been told they would never be able to walk have become able to as the result of acupuncture treatments. Significant improvement is usually apparent by the time ten treatments have been given, but many more treatments may be needed for maximum benefit.

Most children object to needle insertion at first but become very cooperative after they discover that it is not very painful and is helping them control their muscles. Acupuncture is apparently the most effective and safest treatment for cerebral palsy.

Points for treatment include:

Meridian points: Co 4, 10, 11, and 15 · St 36 · UB 23 · Ki 1 and 3 GB 31, 34, and 39 · Br 14

Auricular points: Brain · Lung · Liver · Neck · Thoracic · Lumbar · Sacral · Stomach · Colon

PARALYSIS AND PARESIS

Paralysis is the inability to move a part of the body. Paresis is partial paralysis. Both conditions may be caused by injuries to the nervous system, strokes, or neurologic diseases. Paralysis and paresis may be accompanied by spasticity—involuntary movement which is uncontrollable.

Injuries to the brain and spinal cord from automobile accidents and athletics are common causes of paralysis and paresis. If the spinal cord or any nerve is completely severed, acupuncture cannot correct the paralysis. If the cord or nerve is only damaged, however, acupuncture can improve its functioning and often relieve the resulting paralysis, paresis, and spasticity, even as much as five years after the injury.

Pressure on nerves from spinal disc pathology, arthritis, or vertebral compression from osteoporosis may cause symptoms of paralysis or paresis which can usually be relieved by acupuncture. Sciatic nerve paralysis from buttocks injections can also be relieved by acupuncture. Paralysis caused by such progressive neurologic diseases as multiple sclerosis and amyotrophic lateral sclerosis can be effectively treated by acupuncture but may tend to recur and require a series of treatments several times a year.

Restoring function usually requires many more acupuncture treatments than relieving pain. Some restoration of function may appear after the first few treatments, but many more treatments may be required to obtain optimal function of a limb which has been paralyzed. Nutritional therapy and physical therapy can be given along with acupuncture.

Selection of acupuncture points for treating paralysis and paresis depends on the parts of the body involved. Points for various parts of the body include the following:

Diaphragm

> Meridian points: UB 17 · Li 14 · Sx 15
>
> Auricular points: Diaphragm · Lung · Thoracic

Abdominal muscles

> Meridian points: UB 20 and 21 · St 21 and 25
>
> Auricular points: Abdomen · Thoracic · Diaphragm · Lung · Hip

Upper extremities

> Meridian points: Ex 17 · Co 4, 6, and 11 · Me 5
>
> Auricular points: Shoulder · Elbow · Fingers · Neck

Lower extremities

> Meridian points: Ex 21 · GB 30 and 34 · UB 40 · Li 8 · St 36, 37, and 41 · Ki 3 · Sp 6
>
> Auricular points: Lumbar · Sacral · Hip · Knee · Ankle · Toes

Urethral and rectal sphincters

> Meridian points: Sx 4 · UB 32 and 54

STROKE RESIDUALS

People who survive cerebral hemorrhage or thrombosis usually have some residual disability, such as hemiplegia or aphasia. Function may be partially restored during the first few months afterward, and various techniques of physical medicine and rehabilitation therapy may be helpful.

Most people seeking acupuncture for stroke residuals have had, or are currently having, various types of physiotherapy and occupational therapy which should be continued. Many stroke victims, however, feel they have already derived maximum benefit from these techniques and are reluctant to continue unless they can see some improvement in function.

Acupuncture therapy for stroke residuals is based on the nature and location of the disability. Following is a list of residuals and some of the points used in treating them.

Aphasia, alexia, apraxia, and asteriognosis

Meridian points: Co 4 · St 6 · Sx 14 and 23

Paralysis or partial paralysis of the arms

Meridian points: Co 4, 10, 11, and 15 · Br 15

Paralysis or partial paralysis of the legs

Meridian points: St 36 · UB 23 · Ki 3 · GB 30, 31, 34, and 39

The points for relieving unconsciousness, aphasia, apraxia, alexia, and asteriognosis should be used bilaterally. Paralysis of extremities should be treated with more needles on the paralyzed side but also a few needles on the opposite extremity. Not all points need to be used for each treatment. Points for treating depression and other symptoms should be added when appropriate. Most people who have had strokes feel depressed and frightened, even though they may try to seem cheerful and hopeful.

Electropotentiation of some needles on the afflicted extremity may be useful, but heat is not usually indicated. Paralysis is often accompanied by loss of heat perception. Care should be taken never to burn a patient.

Many stroke victims will notice significant improvement after a few treatments, but usually many months of treatment are required to obtain maximum benefit from acupuncture treatment of stroke residuals.

DYSKINESIA

Dyskinesia is a neurologic disorder caused by medications which damage the basal ganglia of the brain. These include tranquilizers, such as Thorazine, Stelazine, Mellaril, Haldol, Navane, and Prolixin.

The symptoms of this iatrogenic disorder include muscle rigidity and weakness (akinesia), a coarse tremor characteristic of Parkinsonism, uncontrollable restlessness (akathisia), muscular incoordination (dystonia), tics, grimaces, dysarthria, opisthotonos, and torticollis. Physicians should consider the seriousness and discomfort of these symptoms before prescribing psychotropic drugs supposedly to promote relaxation. Most patients taking standard doses of these drugs for a long period of time develop some symptoms of dyskinesia. Some patients develop severe dyskinesia after the first few doses. Acupuncture is more effective and much safer than these drugs for treating mental illness.

In some cases, dyskinesia is relieved simply by discontinuing the drug which caused it. Many cases of dyskinesia, however, persist long after the drug is discontinued. The so-called anti-Parkinsonian drugs, such as Artane, may suppress the symptoms of dyskinesia somewhat but do not protect or heal the basal ganglia of the brain. They produce such side effects as blurred vision, confusion, and hallucinations.

Acupuncture is a safe and effective treatment for dyskinesia. Points for treating it include:

Meridian points: Lu 5 · Co 4, 11, and 15 · St 23 · UB 60 · He 3 · Va 3 and 7 · Me 3 · Sp 6 · Li 3 · GB 30 and 39 · Ki 3 · Br 20 and 24

Auricular points: Brain · Liver · Kidney

PARKINSONISM

Parkinsonism is a neurological disorder characterized by tremor, dyskinesia, rigidity, and deficiency of facial expression. The symptoms may involve only one side of the body at first, but gradually both sides are affected, producing speech impairment and a shuffling unsteady gait with the arms flexed and the hands making involuntary pill-rolling movements. The mind usually remains clear, but the patient tends to become depressed about his situation.

Until the introduction of psychotropic drugs, especially pheno-thiazines, Parkinsonism was seldom seen in people less than 50 years old and was considered to be a delayed result of encephalitis or cerebral arteriosclerosis. Now this syndrome is frequently seen in people of any age who take such drugs as Thorazine and Mellaril which damage the basal ganglia of the brain.

Drugs such as Artane and antihistamines may be somewhat effective in relieving symptoms but have undesirable side effects and tend to become less effective the longer they are taken, especially if the brain-damaging tranquilizers are continued. L-Dopa may be more effective than other drugs in relieving symptoms, but it has worse side effects.

Surgery that destroys various parts of the brain, such as the thalamic nuclei or globus pallidus, has been attempted but has often done more harm than good. Many people have died or become paralyzed and speechless as the result of brain surgery for Parkinsonism.

Acupuncture seems to be the safest and most effective treatment for Parkinsonism. Most patients demonstrate significant improvement in coordination and reduction of tremor by the time they have had ten treatments. For severe or long-standing cases, many more treatments may be indicated. To maintain remission of symptoms, some patients need a series of ten treatments every three or four months.

Standard points include:

Meridian points: Co 4, 11, and 15 · Lu 5 · St 33 · Sp 6 · UB 60 · SI 8 · He 3 · Me 3 · Va 3 and 7 · Ki 3 · GB 30 and 40 · Li 3 · Br 20 and 24

Auricular points: Brain · Liver · Kidney · Neck · Thoracic

All psychotropic and "anti-Parkinsonism" drugs should be discontinued. Acupuncture can treat depression and other emotional problems at the same time the Parkinsonism is being treated. Acupuncture may be more effective than drugs even for schizophrenia. Psychotherapy can be given along with acupuncture.

Patients should have a high protein, low carbohydrate diet and adequate amounts of essential vitamins and minerals, such as Vitamins B1, B2, B6, C, and E; Niacinamide; Biotin; Pantothenate; Calcium; and Zinc.

TREMORS

Tremors are involuntary movements in one or more parts of the body produced by rhythmical alternate contractions of opposing muscle groups. They may be produced by diseases such as Parkinsonism, multiple sclerosis, Wilson's disease, Friedreich's ataxia, arteriosclerosis, or neurosyphilis. Alcohol and narcotic withdrawal may cause tremors temporarily. Psychotropic drugs, such as Thorazine, may cause tremors which persist long after the drug is discontinued. There are also people with a benign hereditary tremor which becomes more pronounced when they are emotionally disturbed.

Since there are so many different causes of tremors, it is important to make the correct diagnosis, especially in the case of alcohol or drug-related tremors. Withdrawal of drugs should be medically supervised, and any therapeutic treatment available should be given before acupuncture.

Acupuncture can relieve tremors from many different causes. It can free patients from drugs, such as L-Dopa and Artane, which have dangerous side effects. Most patients notice considerable reduction in tremor by the time they have had six treatments, but many more treatments may be required for progressive neurologic disorders. Nutritional therapy should be given along with acupuncture and should be discussed with physicians.

Acupuncture points for reducing tremors include:

Meridian points:	St 4 and 6 · UB 1 and 2 · Me 21 and 23 · Sp 6 · SI 18 · Sx 24 · Br 26 · GB 2
Auricular points:	Brain · Liver · Kidney · Neck · Thoracic

ATAXIA

Ataxia is impaired coordination of voluntary muscular action, especially the groups of muscles used for walking or reaching for objects with the hands. A person suffering from ataxia has difficulty maintaining his balance. It is caused by pathology of central or peripheral nervous system pathways involved in balancing muscle movements.

Ingesting alcohol or other drugs can cause temporary ataxia, but ataxia which persists for more than 24 hours after the last dose of an intoxicant requires thorough diagnostic evaluation. Prolonged alcoholism can cause persistent ataxia with cerebellar degeneration, which may be somewhat relieved by megavitamin therapy and acupuncture.

Meniere's disease of the inner ear may cause ataxia along with deafness and/or tinnitus. This can be treated with antibiotics. Multiple sclerosis is a common cause of ataxia which often responds to acupuncture treatments. Brain tumor as a possible cause of ataxia, however, should be carefully ruled out or treated surgically before acupuncture is considered. Pernicious anemia is another possible cause of ataxia which should be diagnosed and treated before acupuncture is given. Diagnosis of the cause of ataxia should never be neglected or delayed because specific treatment for it may be available and more effective if initiated promptly. Acupuncture should not be used to treat tumors such as acoustic neuroma, or to treat anemia or malnutrition, but it can be effective in relieving the symptom of ataxia.

Acupuncture may produce significant improvement in coordination by the time a patient has had six to ten treatments. In many cases, such as multiple sclerosis or other progressive neurologic diseases, several courses of six to ten treatments may bring continuing improvement. Some patients benefit from weekly or monthly maintenance treatments.

The acupuncture points for treating ataxia are generally used bilaterally and may be potentiated by electric stimulation of 30–60 microamperes. The needles are usually left in place 20–30 minutes. The points most frequently used are:

With the patient in a prone position

> Meridian points: UB 8 · GB 9 and 21 · Br 14, 17, and 19 · Me 11 · SI 15 · Ki 6 and 10

With the patient in a supine position

> Meridian points: Br 24 · GB 14 · Li 14 · He 2 · Lu 6 · Ki 26 · Sp 12 · St 36, 40, 41, and 44

> Auricular points: Brain · Kidney · Inner Ear · Liver · Lumbar · Sacral

INCONTINENCE

Incontinence of feces and urine may result from various neurologic disorders, including multiple sclerosis, stroke residuals, spinal cord injuries and tumors, cerebral arteriosclerosis, and brain tumors. It is a difficult problem for the people giving physical care to a patient and very embarrassing to the patient himself.

In many cases acupuncture can improve a person's control of urination and defecation. The points used for incontinence include:

> Meridian points: Co 4 · St 36 · Sp 6 · UB 23 · Sx 2 and 4 · Br 4 and 27

> Auricular points: Brain · Kidney · Lumbar · Sacral · Rectum · Urethra · Urinary Bladder

Sometimes incontinence is relieved after the first or second treatment, but as many as ten treatments are usually required.

MINIMAL BRAIN DYSFUNCTION (HYPERACTIVITY)

A behavior pattern in children characterized by excessive activity, inability to concentrate, and clumsiness is becoming increasingly common in the United States. Although some children do show temporary improvement in their behavior from the amphetamines or Ritalin routinely prescribed for this condition, these drugs are seriously addicting, increase the incidence of strokes in teenagers and are popularly called "speed" when they are obtained illegally.

Minimal brain dysfunction (MBD) is considered to be the cause of this syndrome. Research has indicated that such things as chemical anesthesia given to mothers for childbirth, artificial food colorings and preservatives, drugs taken by pregnant women, and malnutrition may produce brain dysfunction in children. Acupuncture as anesthesia for childbirth reduces the incidence of this disorder.

Acupuncture is a more effective and much safer treatment for hyperactive children than any drug. Although children may not be very cooperative with their first acupuncture treatment, they apparently feel so much better afterwards that they become very willing to have more. Six to ten treatments can give lasting relief from this syndrome in most cases.

All drugs should be discontinued under medical supervision to prevent withdrawal symptoms. Nutrition should be improved by increasing proteins, raw vegetables, and fruit in the diet and by eliminating "junk foods." Certain vitamins may be helpful.

Points for treating MBD include:

Meridian points: Lu 4 · Co 11 · St 36 and 40 · Sp 4 · Va 6 · He 5 · GB 21 · Sx 4 · UB 17, 18, and 20

Auricular points: Brain · Neck · Sympathy

PAIN SYNDROMES

Pain is one of nature's earliest warnings of disease. There are relatively few maladies which do not involve pain. Most people seek medical help primarily because they have pain.

Pain is now regarded as a sensation that depends on its own specific sensory apparatus. The receptors in the skin and deep structures are fine, freely branching nerve endings which form an intricate network. A single primary pain neuron with its cell body in the posterior root ganglion subdivides into many small peripheral branches to supply an area of skin of at least several square millimeters. The cutaneous area of each neuron overlaps with those of other neurons so that each area of skin is within the domain of two to four sensory neurons.

The sensory nerve fibers for pain course through the entire body and are accompanied by motor fibers. They enter the spinal cord and brain stem through the posterior roots and the cranial nerves respectively. The nerve fibers are of two sizes, one very small with a slow conducting velocity, the other somewhat larger with more rapid transmission rates. As the posterior root fibers enter the spinal cord, they terminate in the posterior horn of gray matter. There they synapse with the secondary sensory neuron, the axone of which ascends and crosses the anterior commissure of the spinal cord within three to four segments to find its place in the anterolateral spinothalamic tract. The anterolateral spinothalamic tract continues upward to the posterolateral nucleus of the thalamus in the brain. This tract lies in the anterior part of the spinal cord and passes through the retro-olivary part of the medulla and the dorsolateral parts of the pons and the midbrain. There appears to be a great diminution in the number of fibers as the tract ascends, which means that many of the ascending fibers are terminating in structures located in the brain stem. The thalamic termination of the spinothalamic tracts and the secondary trigeminothalamic tracts, synapse with the third sensory neurons which project to the cortex in the parietal lobes of the brain.

The pain-sensitive structures in the viscera and skin of the body, the mechanisms of their stimulation, and the peripheral nervous pathways are now fairly well established. The skin and mucous membranes, as well as many mesodermal tissues, are sensitive to pain. Despite scientific knowledge of these factors, however, it is often difficult to differentiate between organically and emotionally generated pain. Both factors potentiate each other.

When pain originates in a viscus or deep skeletal tissue, the sensorium recognizes and localizes the pain as arising not from the specific anatomic site involved but from any or all structures innervated by cord segments subserving the affected viscus or deep somatic tissue. The pain appears to be projected toward the body surfaces supplied by these segments.

Any pain is dependent on the brain for perception, and psychological aspects of this phenomenon are significant. It is common knowledge that some individuals are relatively stoical and that others are excessively responsive to pain.

Continuous pain has been observed to have an adverse effect on the entire nervous system, resulting in symptoms of fatigue, insomnia, depression, increased irritability, poor appetite, sexual impotence, and loss of emotional stability. Patients with chronic pain may become irrational about their illnesses and make unreasonable demands. When coupled with the additional deleterious effect of long-term narcotic use, the state which has been termed "pain shock" requires skillful treatment. The choice between giving enough narcotics and other drugs to relieve pain or persuading the patient to tolerate pain without the relief of analgesics was difficult for physicians before acupuncture was available, especially because patients' demands for narcotics tend to increase until dangerously high doses are required or become ineffective.

Before prescribing anything to relieve a patient's pain, the physician should of course regard the pain as a warning signal and diagnose its cause. All physicians know that it is a mistake to relieve pain and thereby mask an important symptom of an ailment which should be promptly treated. After thorough diagnosis and appropriate treatment, however, there is no good reason to let a patient suffer if safe analgesia is available. Acupuncture for temporary pain relief can even be used before diagnosis is completed if pain is severe.

Acupuncture is often more effective than drugs for relieving any type of pain, even the pain of terminal cancer. In the hands of a competent acupuncturist, it is safer than any drug and does not affect the patient's level of consciousness. It enables the patient to be conscious and cooperative while diagnostic studies or surgery are being performed.

Many pains are relieved during the first acupuncture treatment. For lasting relief of pain, however, six treatments are usually required. In most cases, 6–10 needles are inserted at each treatment. Points for depression, insomnia, anxiety, and narcotic addiction are often indicated along with those for pain relief. Electric potentiation is usually beneficial. Pain from progressive diseases, such as metastatic cancer, may require a series of acupuncture treatments every few months or even weeks, but many types of pain are relieved for years after just one series.

Pain in specific areas and from specific causes should be treated with the points indicated under the ailments and areas listed under the appropriate headings. The general points for relieving pain are:

Meridian points: St 36 • Co 4, 11, and 15 • UB 23 and 54 • GB 30, 34, and 54 • Br 14

Auricular points: Brain • Shenmen • Sympathy • Thoracic • Lumbar • Sacral • Neck

Neuralgia and Neuritis

Neuralgia is sharp, stabbing, paroxysmal pain along the course of a nerve. It may not be associated with demonstrable structural changes in the nerve, but there is usually an area of tenderness over the peripheral terminal of the nerve which may be a trigger zone. Even a light touch or temperature change in such areas may initiate a severe attack of the pain. The trigeminal nerve supplying the face may become involved in a neuralgia called "tic douloureux," which often persists for years despite medication and surgical treatment. Other nerves may become similarly involved and resistant to treatment.

Tegretol and other drugs prescribed for neuralgia have potentially lethal side effects and relieve the pain only temporarily if at all. Surgical procedures are hazardous and may result in paralysis of facial or other muscles.

Neuritis is a lesion of nerve tissue and is degenerative or inflammatory. This may cause pain, hypersensitivity, numbness, paresthesia, paralysis, or muscular atrophy. It may be caused by metabolic disorders, such as diabetes or pernicious anemia. Such conditions should be diagnosed and treated before acupuncture is used.

Acupuncture is a safe and effective treatment for both neuralgia and neuritis. It should be accompanied by appropriate nutritional treatment prescribed by supervising physicians. Point selection depends on the area of symptoms. For cephalalgia, see the section on headache. For causalgia, intercostal neuralgia, trigeminal neuralgia (tic douloureux) and sciatic neuralgia (sciatica), see those headings. For points to relieve pain from neuritis or neuralgia in other parts of the body, see those listed in Chapter 13 for analgesia of various parts of the body.

CAUSALGIA

Causalgia is characterized by persistent, diffuse burning pain which tends to recur from various stimuli, such as contact with air or drying of the skin. It is caused by the irritation or injury of a peripheral nerve. The pain may be severe and accompanied by circulatory disturbances, discoloration, coldness, and excessive sweating of the involved part. The muscles of an involved arm or leg may atrophy from immobilization to avoid pain.

There is no effective drug for curing causalgia, but some drugs may relieve the pain for a few hours. Most of these drugs have undesirable side effects and are addictive.

Acupuncture has been very successful in giving lasting relief from the pain of causalgia. When the pain is relieved, the patient is able to use the involved part normally and thereby reduce the other symptoms of this condition.

Improving nutrition will speed recovery from all the symptoms of causalgia. Daily intake of the following nutrients are recommended: Vitamin A (20,000 units), B1 (30 mg.), B2 (30 mg.), B6 (30 mg.), Pantothenic acid (200 mg.), Vitamin C (2 gm.), E (400 units) and Calcium (200 mg.).

As pain is relieved, mild exercise of the involved part should begin. It is important to avoid chilling and medications which may be neurotoxic, such as tranquilizers.

Standard acupuncture points for causalgia include:

Meridian points: Co 11 · Va 5 · Me 6 · St 25 and 29 · Sp 14 and 15

For upper extremities

Auricular points: Neck · Shoulder · Elbow · Fingers

For lower extremities

Auricular points: Lumbar · Hip   Knee · Ankle · Toes

INTERCOSTAL NEURALGIA

Sharp, stabbing pains in the chest between the ribs may make a person think he is having a heart attack, especially if these pains are on the left side. Breathing deeply may be painful. Even though intercostal neuralgia is the most likely cause of such pain, appropriate tests should be done to rule out heart disease.

Another cause of chest pain which may restrict breathing is pleurodynia, which may be a residual of a viral or other infection of the pleura. This condition usually responds well to acupuncture treatment using points similar to those for intercostal neuralgia.

Intercostal neuralgia is caused by inflammation or irritation of the intercostal nerves between the ribs. It may occur infrequently and last only a few seconds without becoming a significant problem. In some cases, however, the episodes of pain recur frequently and last for long periods of time. Acupuncture is usually effective for relieving this type of pain. Six treatments should be given for lasting relief. The points to use include:

Meridian points: Co 11 · Va 5 · Me 6 · GB 38 and 43 · Li 2

Auricular points: Neck · Thoracic · Lumbar · Diaphragm · Lung

Points to relieve anxiety may help to quell a patient's fears that heart disease is present and is so serious that the doctors haven't told him about it. Verbal reassurance may also be helpful.

SCIATIC NEURALGIA (SCIATICA)

Sciatica is painful inflammation of the sciatic nerve. This nerve comes from the fourth and fifth lumbar, and first and second sacral, spinal roots. It provides the motor innervation of the long muscles of the posterior thigh and all the leg muscles below the knee. It transmits sensations from the posterior thigh and side of the leg down to and including the sole of the foot.

Lumbar disc damage and arthritis are the most common causes of sciatica. Other causes include nerve damage from buttocks injections, neurotoxic drugs, metastatic lesions and injuries from trauma.

Drugs with dangerous side effects may relieve the pain temporarily but have no therapeutic effect. Traction with bed rest may relieve the pain by taking pressure off the nerve, but such inactivity encourages the development of thrombosis, which may lead to pulmonary embolism, strokes, and heart attacks. Spinal surgery may relieve or aggravate the symptoms but is hazardous and usually unnecessary unless a tumor is present.

Acupuncture is a safe and effective treatment for sciatica. The pain is usually relieved after the first few treatments. Six to ten treatments are enough for lasting relief in most cases. Large doses of Vitamin C, Pantothenate, Calcium, and Vitamins B1, B6, and B12 can potentiate the effectiveness of acupuncture.

Acupuncture points include:

Meridian points: St 36 · UB 23, 25, 31, 49, 50, 54, and 60 · GB 34 and 39 · Br 25

Auricular points: Lumbar · Sacral · Shenmen · Sympathy

TRIGEMINAL NEURALGIA (Tic Douloureux)

Trigeminal neuralgia is a syndrome manifested by episodes of brief but severe pain along one or more distributions of the trigeminal (fifth cranial) nerve. Although at times associated with atherosclerosis, the disease process is usually unassociated with detectable organic lesions in the trigeminal nerve, and its etiology remains unknown. It tends to afflict women slightly more frequently than men, with the sixth decade of life being the usual time the symptoms appear.

The maxillary (second division) and mandibular (third division) branches are most commonly involved. Early in the disease process, attacks are short (one to two minutes in duration) and infrequent with asymptomatic periods up to several months between them. As the disease advances, however, the attacks last longer and become more frequent. In extreme cases, hypersensitive areas on the face known as trigger points exist. These trigger points, when subjected to light tactile stimulation (such as shaving, brushing the teeth, talking, or eating), are capable of initiating a full-blown attack of trigeminal neuralgia.

The diagnosis of trigeminal neuralgia is made by its typical history and the distribution of pain. Post-herpetic neuralgia (shingles) can mimic trigeminal neuralgia. The evidence of a cutaneous eruption associated with a history of precedent herpes zoster, however, usually establishes the diagnosis of post-herpetic neuralgia.

The treatment of trigeminal neuralgia is both medical and surgical, but neither is very safe or effective in most cases. Medical management entails the use of various analgesics, carbamazepine (Tegretol), or diphenylhydantoin (Dilantin). The adverse reactions or undesirable side effects of these drugs, however, can be extremely serious or even fatal. It is unfortunate that most physicians do not warn their patients about these before prescribing them.

Aspirin, and the many well-advertised brands of analgesics containing this drug, increase a person's tendency to bleed and bruise. It is also irritating to the stomach and likely to cause ulcers. Bleeding gums are a frequent result of prolonged aspirin therapy. Severe anemia can be produced by aspirin with bleeding from various internal organs.

Codeine, Methadone, Demerol, and other narcotics are addictive. Increasing doses are required for pain relief until the lethal dose is approached. Gradual withdrawal from narcotics is difficult. Sudden withdrawal can produce serious and very unpleasant symptoms.

Dilantin is a drug usually given to control convulsive disorders. Attempts at intravenous injection can be very irritating to surrounding tissues because of the high alkalinity of the drug. Intravenous injection can produce severe hypoglycemia, causing convulsions, respiratory depression, anoxia, and shock. Giving Dilantin orally is safer, but adverse reactions to it may be serious.

Tegretol may suppress the bone marrow and cause aplastic

anemia or agranulocytosis. It may also cause urinary retention, sexual impotence, atrophy of the testicles, dizziness, blurred vision, hallucinations, tinnitus, and heart failure.

Surgical therapy includes 98% alcohol injection into the involved branch of the trigeminal nerve as it exits from its cranial foramina or insertion of a piece of plastic. These techniques involve the hazards of brain surgery but have resulted in remission for as long as 24 months. Peripheral nerve avulsion (cutting the involved branch at its exit from the skull) has resulted in palliation ranging between 9 and 24 months. Permanent relief may be obtained by sectioning the sensory root of the trigeminal nerve proximal to the Gasserian ganglion (trigeminal rhizotomy, gangliolysis), hopefully with preservation of the motor branch to the muscles of mastication. This latter procedure is usually reserved for cases refractory to less radical measures since it carries with it the inherent risks and morbidity associated with entering the skull and the possibility of facial paralysis.

Some patients have their teeth pulled in a desperate effort to rid themselves of this excruciating pain, which seems like a severe toothache in some cases, but the pain persists.

Acupuncture has a high rate of success for trigeminal neuralgia and is, of course, safer than drugs or surgery. It has been successful in many cases after surgery has failed to give relief of pain. Usually six to ten treatments give lasting relief.

The points used include:

Meridian points: Co 4, 11, 19, and 20 · St 4, 6, 7, 8, 40, and 44 · UB 2 and 62 · Br 26 · Me 17 and 21 · SI 17, 18, and 19

For mandibular pain, the following points should be included:

Meridian points: GB 3, 14, and 20 · Co 10

Auricular points: Maxillary Sinus · Eye I and II · Upper and Lower Teeth· Forehead· Shenmen · Sympathy

Herpes Zoster (Shingles)

Herpes Zoster is a virus considered to be the same as the one causing chickenpox. After a person has had chickenpox (varicella), usually in childhood, the virus is thought to lie dormant in his body until years later. When he is in a weakened condition (from malnutrition, other infection, injury, or emotional strain), it attacks a dorsal nerve root.

The trigeminal nerve supplying the face and the thoracic nerves are the ones usually involved but only on one side of the body.

The first symptom is pain in the involved area. Then pustules similar to those of chickenpox appear there. Recovery may be almost complete within a month for people who are in general good health, but some, especially elderly people who have debilitating diseases, may continue to have severe nerve root pain for years, perhaps the rest of their lives.

No drug has been found effective for this condition. Some that have been prescribed by physicians have done more harm than good. Certain nutrients seem to be helpful. These are: Vitamins B1 (20 mg.), B2 (20 mg.), B6 (20 mg.), Pantothenic acid (200 mg.), C (2 gm.), D (800 units), E (400 units), and Calcium (200 mg.) daily.

Acupuncture can greatly reduce the severity of herpes zoster symptoms and relieve persistent residual pain. Narcotics may be required to relieve pain until after the first few acupuncture treatments. The pain is usually gone by the time a patient has had six acupuncture treatments.

Acupuncture points for shingles include:

Meridian points: Co 4 and 11 · Sp 6 and 10 · UB 11–14, 21, and 22

For facial lesions

Meridian points: GB 1 and 2 · SI 19 · St 1 · Me 23

Auricular points: Forehead · Eye I and II

For lesions of the thorax

Meridian points: UB 15–20 · GB 24 and 25 · St 20–25 · Sp 16 · Li 14 and 16 on the opposite side.

Auricular points: Thoracic · Shenmen · Sympathy

Headache

Pain in the head may arise in the pain-sensitive structures within the cranium (meninges and large arteries) or in the extracranial tissues of the head and neck (occipital, temporal, and frontal muscle groups, the skin of the scalp, and the extracranial arteries). Types of headache include sinus, migraine, thalamic, cluster, hypertensive, hypoglycemic, tension, brain tumor, and temporal arteritis. The latter two require surgery and should not be treated by acupuncture.

One of the commonest types of headache is the tension headache. It is usually occipital in location but may occasionally be frontal. Such headaches can be identified by their relationship to emotional stress or fatigue and are often accompanied by tenderness of the posterior neck muscles. The headaches of eye strain may be present with similar symptoms, but the cause is usually readily identifiable. Headaches described as being "like a sense of pressure" or like a "tight constricting band" are usually classified as tension headaches.

Migraine headaches may have an allergic and/or familial component. They usually involve only one side of the head and may be accompanied by nausea, dizziness, and visual distortions. Some people refer to these as "histamine headaches" and attempt to treat them by antihistamine drugs or desensitization to histamine. The results of such treatment, however, are usually disappointing.

Many patients with severe headaches have been given narcotic preparations, such as codeine and demerol, or aspirin for temporary relief. Belladona alkaloids and ergotamine (Cafergot) are frequently prescribed. If these are ineffective, dimethysergide (Sansert) may be used. All of these drugs have unacceptable side effects and are not recommended for long-term use. Even aspirin can cause stomach ulcers and bruising. Acetaminophen (Datril and Tylenol) do not upset the stomach but can cause liver damage. Demerol and codeine are narcotics that may cause addiction. Caffeine irritates the heart muscle and can cause palpitation as well as anxiety and insomnia. Ergot derivatives constrict the peripheral blood vessels and can cause hypertension and other circulatory problems. An overdose can lead to gangrene, requiring amputation of the limbs. Methysergide causes fibrosis of the lungs, heart valves, major blood vessels, and other vital organs. It can also cause hair loss, edema, and hallucinations.

Most patients obtain lasting relief of headaches after six acupuncture treatments. Some require more treatments or a series of six treatments as often as every six months. Since there is no drug that is safe as well as effective for relieving headaches, acupuncture should be considered the treatment of choice.

The classical points for treating headache include:

Meridian points: Lu 7 · Co 4 · St 8, 29, 30, 36, 40, and 43 · Sp 5, 6, 8, and 9 · UB 2, 7, 23, 25, and 62 · Ki 1 and 3 · Me 4, 6, 15, and 23 · GB 4, 5, 7, 20, and 40 · Li 1, 2, 3, and 8 · Sx 6 · Br 16, 19, 20, and 23.

Six to twenty needles should be inserted for each treatment. Electric or infrared heat potentiation are usually unnecessary.

Accidents: Emergency Relief of Pain from Trauma

Acupuncture is safer than chemical analgesics for relieving pain in emergencies before a definitive diagnosis can be made. It does not alter the level of consciousness or cause allergic reactions. Although it can greatly reduce the degree of pain, it does not cause the numbness associated with local anesthetics and is, therefore, much less likely to mask symptoms. The patient continues to be aware of where his pain is but does not feel it intensely. Acupuncture can also reduce a patient's fear, anxiety, apprehensiveness, and nausea after an injury. It can promote homeostasis and thus avoid shock, which is often a serious complication of accidental injuries.

Ambulance and other paramedical personnel could relieve much unnecessary suffering and probably save some lives if they were able to give prompt pain and anxiety relief with acupuncture. Acupuncture charts and handbooks should be carried in all ambulances along with sterilized acupuncture needles.

The acupuncture points to use for relieving pain in an emergency situation depend on the location of the pain and are as follows:

Abdomen

Meridian points: St 36 and 39 · Sp 6 · Li 3 · Br 4 · GB 28 and 34 · Me 6

Auricular points: Abdomen · Lung · Sympathy

Anxiety, apprehensiveness

Meridian points: GB 20 · UB 15 and 19 · He 5 and 7 · Lu 4 · Va 4 (for treating shock)

Auricular points: Shenmen · Sympathy · Liver

Arms

Meridian points: Co 11, 12, and 15 · GB 34 · Me 5

Auricular points: Fingers · Elbow · Shoulder

Chest

Meridian points: Co 3 and 4 · Va 4 and 6 · Me 5 and 8 · GB 34 · UB 65

Auricular points: Shenmen · Lung · Kidney · Thoracic · Spleen · Diaphragm

Ears

Meridian points: Co 4 · Me 3 and 17 · Va 3 · GB 43

Eyes

Meridian points: Co 4 · St 2 · GB 14 and 20 · Me 5

Auricular points: Shenmen · Lung · Eye II

Head

Meridian points: SI 18 · Li 3 · St 43 · GB 8 and 41 · UB 2

Auricular points: Internal Nose · Brain · Inner Ear

Hips

Meridian points: St 36 and 40 · UB 59 · GB 30, 36, and 39 · Sp 6 · Li 5

Auricular points: Hip · Lumbar

Legs

Meridian points: GB 30, 34, and 39 · St 35

Auricular points: Knee · Ankle

Lumbar and Pelvic

Meridian points: UB 23 and 40 · SI 3 and 6 · Br 26

Auricular points: Urinary Bladder · Lumbar · Urethra · Rectum · Colon · Uterus

Mouth

Meridian points: Co 4 · St 5–7, and 44 · Me 21

Auricular points: Upper and Lower Teeth · Pharynx

Nausea

Meridian points: Va 6 · St 36

Auricular points: Stomach · Liver · Sympathy

Neck

Meridian points: Co 4 · St 6 and 44 · Va 6 · GB 20 and 39 · SI 6

Nose

Meridian points: Co 4 and 20 · St 2 · Br 24

Auricular points: Pharynx · Internal Nose · External Nose · Maxillary Sinus · Lung

Shoulder

Meridian points: St 38 · UB 57 · Co 11, 15, and 16 · SI 10 · GB 34 · Me 14

Auricular points: Neck · Shoulder · Shenmen · Sympathy

Throat

Meridian points: Co 4 · St 6 and 44 · Va 6

Auricular points: Pharynx · Larynx · Neck · Lung · Shenmen

chapter 21

PSYCHIATRIC AND EMOTIONAL DISORDERS

Many emotional problems that normal people have at one time or another can be effectively treated by acupuncture while the patient undergoes counseling or psychotherapy or simply tries to ameliorate the circumstances of his life situation himself. Acupuncture can relieve feelings of anxiety and depression, which may be serious handicaps for people trying to cope with difficult domestic, social, and vocational problems. Acupuncture can also relieve insomnia and give a person a feeling of well-being and self-confidence. It is an effective substitute for sleeping pills, tranquilizers, and antidepressant drugs.

There is increasing evidence that many serious psychiatric disorders have an organic basis, possibly metabolic or allergic. Metabolism and allergic reactions are getting more attention from psychiatrists than previously.

Many different attempts at classifying psychiatric and emotional disorders have been made and officially adopted by the medical profession at different times. None of these has been very satisfactory.

Many psychiatrists have questioned whether there actually are any mental diseases. There are, however, recognizable behavior patterns and subjective symptoms which are distressing. In this section, psychiatric and emotional problems and their acupuncture treatment are discussed under the following headings. This classification does not conform to the current classification adopted by the American Psychiatric Association. Sexual problems are discussed in chapter 6 on the genital system.

NEUROSES

Neuroses are inappropriate behavior patterns adopted by sane people to relieve and mask their conscious or unconscious anxiety, depression, and feelings of guilt. These behavior patterns may be recognized as phobias, hypochondriasis, obsessive-compulsive activities and attitudes, paranoid thinking, impulsiveness, insomnia, affective lability, dissociative reactions, persistent sadness, laziness, or conversion hysteria with sensory or sexual dysfunction, paralysis or psychosomatic illness.

Psychotherapy may be helpful in reducing neuroses but may require months, or even years, and be very expensive. In many cases, acupuncture can relieve neurotic symptoms with six to ten treatments. It can be given along with psychotherapy and should be used as a substitute for psychotropic drugs, all of which have undesirable side effects. Besides causing allergic reactions and addictions, psychotropic drugs can cause lasting damage to the nervous system and other parts of the body. The relief of anxiety and depression given by drugs usually lasts only a few hours after medication is discontinued, whereas the relief given by a series of six to ten acupuncture treatments may last for several years.

Six or more points should be used for each treatment. Points for relieving depression and anxiety should be selected in accordance with clinical evaluation of these factors and response. Classical points for anxiety include:

Meridian points: Lu 4 · Co 11 · St 36 and 40 · Sp 4 · He 3, 5, and 7 · UB 15, 17, 18, 19, and 23 · Va 4 · GB 20 and 21 · Sx 4, 9, and 12

Those for depression include:

Meridian points: Lu 5, 7, and 10 · Co 15 · St 25 and 44 · Sp 6 ·
                   He 6 · SI 3 · UB 11, 13, 19, 20, 23, 38, and 60
                   · Ki 6 · Va 5, 6, and 8 · Me 6 · GB 20 · Li 2
Auricular points: Lung · Brain · Sympathy

AFFECTIVE DISORDERS

People with moods of depression alternating with moods of excitement
and hyperactivity are emotionally unstable and may be considered to
have an affective disorder. Such mood alterations may be mild and
related to the circumstances or events of a person's life, or they may
be severe and not obviously related to anything outside the patient's
body. This latter type of mood disturbance is considered abnormal and
usually requires treatment. Sometimes periods of depression or hyperactivity last for months at a time and seriously interfere with a person's job and personal relationships. People with this type of affective
disorder are said to have manic-depressive illness or psychosis.

They do not respond well to electric shock or convulsive treatments and should never be subjected to them. Sedatives may be
required to control extreme hyperactive episodes to prevent the
patient from injuring himself or others. The so-called antidepressants,
however, are usually not very effective and may have serious side
effects. Lithium carbonate has been the most effective drug used for
affective disorders, but it requires daily dosage of the drug and laboratory tests every few weeks to check for toxic effects on the kidneys
and other organs.

Megavitamin therapy and high protein diets contribute to emotional stability and reduce severe mood swings. Large doses of Niacinamide, Vitamin C, Vitamin E, calcium, and zinc are considered the
most important, but the other vitamins and essential minerals should
be given along with them. This type of treatment, combined with acupuncture, is a much safer and more effective way to treat emotional
instability than drugs with side effects or electric shock.

Acupuncture treatments should be given on a daily basis, if possible, until ten treatments have been given. This will often be sufficient
for a patient who stays on a good diet supplemented by vitamins and
does not have a major crisis or continual frustration to cope with in his
life situation. Some patients may require a few more treatments after
several months or years. Others seem to benefit greatly and maintain
their emotional stability by having acupuncture weekly or every two
weeks for several months.

The acupuncture points used to treat emotional instability include the following.

Auricular points: Lung · Brain · Sympathy

To maintain stability:

Meridian points: Br 12, 13, 14, 16, and 23 · Lu 7 and 9 · St 37 · Co 9 · Va 4 and 5 · He 7 · Li 1 · Sx 12 and 15

For the hyperactive phase, the following points are especially helpful:

Meridian points: Sp 1 and 6 · Lu 5 and 11 · Sx 14 and 24 · St 6 and 36 · Br 16

For the depressive phase, the following points bring relief most promptly:

Meridian points: Li 3 · Co 4 and 11 · Va 7 · Lu 7 · Br 16 and 20 · He 7 · UB 62 · GB 14 and 34 · Ki 6 · St 8 and 45

The points for insomnia and anxiety can also be used.

Depression

Depression is both a cause and result of chronic illness. Most chronically ill people are depressed, but it is not always possible to determine whether they became ill because they were depressed or became depressed because of their illness. Physicians should be perceptive of signs of depression in their patients and treat depression along with other medical problems. But not all depressed people consider themselves sick.

There are basically two types of depression—exogenous and endogenous. Exogenous depression results from factors in the external environment, such as loss of a loved one. Endogenous depression is caused by factors within the person's body and may be independent of his life situation.

Some researchers have found deficiencies of the biochemicals serotonin and dopamine in depressed patients and have, therefore, concluded that endogenous depression is a symptom of biochemical deficiency which can be corrected by drugs. As a result, many drugs have been developed to treat depression. Most of these drugs are at least somewhat effective but have serious side effects. It cannot be determined, however, whether the biochemical deficiencies in depression result from the patient's attitude toward life, or whether the bio-chemical deficiencies occur for other reasons and cause the attitudes and thinking patterns characteristic of depression. Taking lithium regularly has proved effective in many cases of depression which are a part of the manic-depressive syndrome, but this drug has caused kidney damage and blood dyscrasia.

Many psychiatrists consider electro-convulsive treatments (sometimes called electric shock treatments) the most effective treatment for depression and a life-saving procedure for many suicidal patients. These treatments cause enough memory loss to make a patient forget what he was depressed about and are, therefore, effective at least temporarily. Even if the memory loss persists, however, the depression will usually recur within a few months. There is no satisfactory scientific explanation of how electro-convulsive therapy relieves depression. Some pathologists have reported evidence of microscopic hemorrhages in the brain tissue of people who have had electro-convulsive therapy. This brain damage, with the consequent impairment of thought processes, seems the most likely explanation of why electro-convulsive therapy is sometimes effective.

Considering the instances of bone fractures from the convulsions, burns at the site of electrode applications, and permanent memory impairment, as well as deaths from apena or cardiac arrest, this traumatic procedure seems inappropriate for acceptance in American medical practice, and its use has gradually declined during the past 20 years. It is less expensive than drugs or psychotherapy and was frequently used by underfunded state mental hospitals and private hospitals as a way of reducing expenses.

Gynecologists and general practitioners have considered depression as part of the menopausal syndrome and, until recently, prescribed female hormones for women past 35 for this reason. Many women, however, have become depressed from taking female hormones for contraceptive purposes. The increase in hormone prescriptions for depression or contraception has coincided with an increased incidence of breast and genital cancer, strokes, and heart attacks in women. This connection between hormone medication and cancer has belatedly been officially recognized by the Food and Drug Administration. There is no valid evidence that female hormones relieve depression. Too many women have had their chances of developing cancer, strokes, and heart attacks increased by physicians who have made the mistake of prescribing hormones to relieve depression.

Acupuncture is a safe and effective way to relieve depression. It will not, of course, change the circumstances of a person's life, but it will usually produce a feeling of well-being and relieve the insomnia which infrequently accompanies depression. In cases of exogenous depression, depression resulting from loss of a loved one, financial problems, chronic illness, or disability, supportive psychotherapy is helpful. As the heavy, sad feeling of depression is relieved, a person feels more confidence in his ability to cope with unpleasant aspects of his life situation and make necessary changes. Acupuncture will not replace the biochemical deficiencies found in some endogenous depressions, but it does promote normalization of body metabolism and stimulates the patient's body to produce optimal amounts of the biochemicals it needs for good health. Since acupuncture does not have the side effects of antidepressant drugs, electric shock, or hormones, it is much safer and usually at least as effective.

Acupuncture treatment for depression can be given along with treatment for any other symptoms. The most commonly used acupuncture points for relieving depression are:

Meridian points: UB 11, 13, 19, 20, 23, 38, and 60 • Co 15 • GB 20 • St 25 and 44 • He 6 • Va 5, 6, and 8 • Sp 6 • Lu 5, 7, and 10 • Me 6 • Ki 6 • Li 2 • SI 3

Six or more of these points should be used for each treatment. They may be potentiated by 50–150 microamperes of pulsating current for 15–30 minutes unless the patient has heart irregularities. Considerable relief from depression is usually experienced after the first treatment, but six treatments should be given to obtain lasting relief.

Anxiety

Anxiety is the restless apprehensiveness which complicates many illnesses and may precede their development. Patients suffering from uncomplicated anxiety may appear acutely ill with dyspnea, tachycardia, hyperhidrosis, prostration, and fear that death is imminent. Hysterical symptoms, such as the paralysis of a limb, inability to speak, hear, or see, may be produced by anxiety. According to theories of psychosomatic medicine, anxiety may be a major cause of such serious pathology as peptic ulcer, ulcerative colitis, bronchial asthma, myocardial infarction, and neurodermatitis. Anxiety usually accompanies pain and intensifies it. Although anxiety is classified as a psychoneurosis and may be a prominent symptom of psychotic episodes, most people have experienced this unpleasant emotion at times. Patients who complain of nervousness and insomnia are generally suffering from anxiety.

Tranquilizing drugs are effective for the temporary relief of anxiety but may have dangerous side effects and are destructive to the basal ganglia of the brain if taken in large doses over a long period of time. Barbiturates and narcotics are effective for relieving anxiety but are addictive and lethal when overdoses are taken. Alcohol is the most readily available drug for relief of anxiety, but the consequences of self-medication with alcohol may be disastrous. Megavitamin therapy is safe and often helpful in treating anxiety. It can be given along with acupuncture and continued afterwards.

Traditional Chinese medicine considers anxiety a symptom of imbalance between the *Yin* and *Yang* aspects of vital energy. In many cases, it can be effectively relieved by acupuncture. The points used for treating anxiety are included in the treatment of many types of illness, especially for the relief of pain which may accompany them.

The points usually used at the Washington Acupuncture Center are:

Meridian points: Co 11 · St 36 · Sp 4 · GB 20 and 21 · Sx 4 and 6 · Br 14 and 20 · UB 15 and 19 · He 3, 5, and 7 · Lu 4

Another combination of points sometimes used is:

Meridian points: UB 15, 17, and 18 · He 7 · Va 4 · Br 4 · Sx 9 and 12 · St 36 and 40

Although acupuncture can relieve the symptoms of anxiety, it should not be considered as a substitute for psychotherapy. Most patients with anxiety are involved in life situations which are threatening and aggravating. They should be encouraged to obtain help for coping with these situations and will usually be more willing to do this after having their symptoms relieved by acupuncture.

How long the relief of anxiety by acupuncture lasts is somewhat dependent on how severe the problems are that the patient must cope with in his daily life. Some patients treated over three years ago have remained essentially free from anxiety symptoms since their first six treatments. Others have returned for more acupuncture treatments every four to six months.

ANOREXIA

Loss of appetite can be a transitory symptom brought on by fear, anger, or grief. In such cases it is not serious and hardly worth treating, but anorexia nervosa is a life-threatening psychosomatic disorder which usually requires psychotherapy and has a poor prognosis. Before assuming that anorexia is purely psychogenic, such factors as malfunctioning viscera or metabolic disorders should be ruled out. Standard treatment for any diagnosed pathology should be given before acupuncture is attempted.

Acupuncture points for anorexia are:

Meridian points: St 36 · UB 18 and 20 · Ki 4

Auricular points: Brain · Stomach · Liver

If a person complains of nausea, Va 6 should be added. If anxiety is evident or suspected, points Lu 4 · He 3, 5, and 7 · UB 15 and 19 and GB 20 might be helpful. In some cases, the acupuncture points for neurasthenia will speed recovery.

Supportive psychotherapy, a nutritious diet which appeals to the patient, and, if necessary, parenteral feeding should be given along with acupuncture.

FATIGUE

Fatigue is excessive tiredness, a feeling that any activity is a tremendous effort. This may be a symptom of heart disease or other serious medical problems and requires a thorough diagnostic evaluation. Most cases of fatigue, however, are not related to disease.

Chinese theory attributes fatigue to an imbalance of body energy which can be corrected by acupuncture treatments. A patient usually begins to feel more energetic after his first acupuncture treatment and will have a normal amount of energy and interest in work by the time he has had six treatments, unless he is suffering from a debilitating disease.

Along with acupuncture, a patient should improve his nutrition by taking the following daily: Vitamin A (10,000 units), B1 (20 mg.), B2 (20 mg.), B6 (20 mg.), Pantothenic acid (200 mg.), Niacinamide (500 mg.), Folic acid (0.4 mg.), B12 (200 mcg.), C (2 gm.), and E (400 units). He should exclude from his diet artificially colored and sweetened foods, candy, cake, pie, cola, chocolate, fried food, and alcohol while increasing his intake of raw fruit, vegetables and proteins, such as eggs, milk, fish, and lean meat. Hypoglycemia from a high carbohydrate, low protein diet is a frequent component of fatigue. Vitamin deficiency is another common cause of fatigue which can be easily corrected.

Emotional causes of fatigue, such as depression, may be relieved by psychotherapy along with acupuncture. Most drugs, even antidepressants, increase fatigue and should be discontinued.

Acupuncture points for treatment of fatigue include:

Meridian points: St 36 • UB 18 and 20 • Ki 2 • Li 2, 3, 4, and 14 • Sx 12

Auricular points: Brain • Liver • Lung

INSOMNIA

Insomnia is difficulty sleeping and is a problem to almost everyone at times. The amount of sleep a person needs depends on many factors which are difficult to identify and analyze, but very few people actually need more than six hours of sleep out of 24 to maintain optimum health. Many people worry unnecessarily because they think they need more sleep than they actually do. In general, older people need less sleep than children, adolescents, or young adults. Some people who have lived long and successful lives have claimed that they seldom slept more than four hours out of 24.

Lack of exercise, worry, fear, anxiety, anger, malnutrition, grief, and pain may cause insomnia. Medications, such as barbiturates and tranquilizers, which are given to promote sleep may actually increase insomnia and cause addiction if taken regularly for even a week. They deprive a person of normal sleep, make him feel depressed during the day after taking them, and may induce muscle spasms. Sudden withdrawal from barbiturates may even cause convulsions.

By relieving pain and anxiety, acupuncture will almost always relieve insomnia. Acupuncture treatment for insomnia can be given along with treatment for other conditions which may be causative factors in insomnia. Some patients begin to sleep well after their first acupuncture treatment, even before symptoms of their other medical problems have been completely relieved. Six acupuncture treatments are usually enough to restore a normal sleep pattern, even in patients who have suffered from insomnia for many years.

Taking a daily supplement of calcium lactate (10 grains), Vitamin C (2 gm.), Thiamin (20 mg.), Pyridoxine (20 mg.) and the essential amino acid L-Tryptophane (1–2 gm. at bedtime) is more effective than taking sleeping pills and eliminates the nutritional causes of insomnia. Deficiencies of these nutrients is a common cause of insomnia. They are available without a prescription and promote general good health. Physicians might also recommend other nutrients and diet changes to help relieve insomnia.

Psychotherapy and counseling about personal problems may be

helpful for relieving worry, fear, anger, resentment, and grief as well as helping a person to change his life style to obtain more exercise, avoid excessive stimulation just before bedtime, and learn how to relax.

Acupuncture points for relieving insomnia include:

Meridian points: Lu 9 • Co 4 and 11 • Sp 4 • He 7 • Ki 1 and 3

Auricular points: Shenmen • Sympathy • Liver • Kidney

Points for relieving snoring and disturbances of breathing during sleep include:

Meridian points: GB 2, 20, and 40 • Br 26 • UB 15 and 18 • SI 19 • Sx 12

Auricular points: Brain • Sympathy • Pharynx • Internal Nose • Lung • Maxillary Sinus • Tonsil

NERVOUSNESS

Almost everyone feels nervous occasionally, but nervousness may be a serious and chronic problem for some people. Such people are often highly intelligent but lack self-confidence and the ability to cope with frustrating situations.

The anxiety symptoms from nervousness may cause blushing, excessive perspiration, palpitation of the heart, shortness of breath, nausea, vomiting, stomach pain, and diarrhea. These symptoms may be very disabling and make a person think he has a serious disease. Such fear produces worry which may keep the nervous person awake at night and may actually impair his physical health.

Acupuncture is very effective for promoting relaxation and relieving all the symptoms of nervousness. Most patients experience a feeling of well-being after the first treatment and usually have lasting relief from nervousness by the time they have had six to ten treatments.

Many drugs for relieving nervousness are advertised on radio and television. Although they are available without a prescription, they may have serious side effects. Prescription drugs for nervousness, such as Thorazine and other tranquilizers, damage the basal ganglia of the brain. There is increasing medical evidence that Valium, Librium, and other "minor tranquilizers" are addictive as well as dangerous. Acupuncture is more effective and safer than any drug for treating nervousness. Points to use include:

Meridian points: Co 11 · St 36 · Sp 4 · Va 6 · GB 21 · Sx 6 · Br
14 and 20

Auricular points: Lung · Brain · Sympathy

SPEECH DISORDERS

Speech disorders, such as stuttering, stammering, aphasia, and hoarseness may respond to acupuncture treatments. In cases of hoarseness, however, laryngeal and other examinations should be made to rule out the possibility of vocal cord tumors or neoplasms of other structures exerting pressure on the larynx.

Although the causes of stuttering and stammering are generally considered to be psychologic, these conditions may respond to acupuncture treatments. Some speech disorders respond slowly. At least ten treatments are usually necessary for significant improvement.

The points used for treating various types of speech disorders include:

Meridian points: Co 4 and 11 · St 6 and 36 · Sp 4 · Va 6 · GB 21
· Sx 6, 14, and 23 · Br 14 and 20

Auricular points: Pharynx · Larynx · Neck · Maxillary Sinus ·
Upper Teeth · Lung · Shenmen · Sympathy

ADDICTIVE DISORDERS

An obsessive craving for excessive amounts of anything may be considered an addictive disorder. Addiction may be physiologic or psychologic, but it is usually both.

Withdrawal symptoms of various types occur when a person attempts to deny himself the substance to which he has become addicted. Even the person who has the habit of eating too much will experience stomach cramps and possibly hypoglycemia if he tries to diet without medical supervision. The withdrawal symptoms from alcoholism may be extremely serious, even fatal. Sudden withdrawal of drugs on which a person has become dependent may be equally serious.

Some drugs, such as Valium, which were considered non-addictive for several years after they were on the market, have recently been recognized as addictive. Cortisone derivatives are still classified as non-addictive, but sudden withdrawal of these drugs can cause an adrenal crisis and death. Although acupuncture can reduce the withdrawal symptoms from narcotics, alcohol, and dieting, it should not be expected to prevent withdrawal symptoms from cortisone derivatives, barbiturates, amphetamines, and some tranquilizing drugs. These must be discontinued gradually.

Drug Dependence

Besides drug dependence on narcotics, barbiturates, or amphetamines, drug dependence on hormone replacements, such as cortisone or estrogen, and various tranquilizers may create serious problems, including withdrawal reactions which can be life-threatening. Some drugs must be reduced gradually under careful medical supervision, while others, such as insulin, must be continued. Acupuncture can be especially helpful in treating drug withdrawal from narcotics and other addictive drugs, but it cannot always be depended on as the only treatment in severe cases.

Besides acupuncture, drug addicts should have psychotherapy and a supportive environment free from drugs. They usually have serious emotional conflicts, which they need to work through, and may also require some counseling about changing their life style. Group therapy has been found effective in treating many addicts, but others are too emotionally fragile to benefit from it.

Since drug addicts usually have poor eating habits, they often suffer from malnutrition which should be treated with a high protein, low carbohydrate diet supplemented by multivitamins and minerals. Vitamin C and the B vitamins Pyridoxine and Niacinamide are especially helpful in relieving the feelings of emptiness and craving that accompany drug addiction.

Because drug addicts tend to drop out of treatment programs, some physicians have inserted surgical staples into the lung points on the ear pinnas, leaving these staples in place for several weeks. This procedure has the advantage of not requiring more than one session with the physician but is not as effective as regular acupuncture treatments.

The acupuncture points used for treating drug addiction are:

Meridian points: St 8, 15, 25, and 40 · Sx 10, 12, 13, and 14 · Br
                   20 · GB 20 and 34 · Ki 1 · Sp 1 and 6 · Va 7 ·
                   He 7 · Lu 7 · SI 3 · Me 6

Auricular points: Lung · Liver · Abdomen

Some or all of these can be potentiated with 30–100 microamperes of pulsating current with a sawtooth or square wave. Treatments can be given twice a day during the withdrawal period and then on a daily or weekly basis until six to ten treatments have been given. Only 6–14 needles should be inserted for each treatment. Usually the effects of treatment last for years, and one course of acupuncture may be adequate to correct the addiction if the patient is not subjected to severe temptation or frustration in his daily life. If the drug problem begins to recur after several months, another course of acupuncture can be given. Patients who have had a serious addiction problem for many years may benefit from acupuncture every week or two for maintenance of their drug-free condition.

Alcoholism

Much has been written about alcoholism, and many theories have been developed about its cause and cure. It is generally agreed that some people are more likely to become alcoholics than others, but identifying potential alcoholics before they begin drinking alcohol is not yet possible. Alcohol is the most readily available tranquilizer. Many people turn to it to relieve emotional or other pain. Few people are willing to admit that they have an alcohol problem until it is far advanced.

Some drugs, such as Valium, which have been given to treat alcoholism have been found to potentiate the effects of alcohol and are addictive themselves. Barbiturates, antidepressants, and other psychotropic drugs also augment the undesirable effects of alcohol and are not indicated in the treatment of alcoholism.

Antabuse is a drug which alcoholics are often given to take each morning with the knowledge that, if they drink even a little alcohol within 24 hours, they will vomit and become seriously ill. Too many people have died from drinking alcohol while on antabuse, sometimes unknowingly. Most cough medicines and food flavorings, for instance, contain alcohol. Most alcoholics have poor health and are not able to tolerate the serious complications caused by ingesting alcohol after antabuse medication.

Withdrawal symptoms when an alcoholic stops thinking for a day or two are called *delirium tremens* and are life-threatening. The fear of these symptoms makes it almost impossible for alcoholics to stop drinking without medical help.

Research on alcoholics has revealed that almost all of them have eaten a high carbohydrate, low protein diet since childhood, which has given them hypoglycemia. Hypoglycemia is a metabolic disorder in which the blood sugar rises steeply after carbohydrate ingestion but within an hour drops precipitously to levels low enough to cause feelings of faintness and disorientation, headache, and depression. Alcohol, a carbohydrate, brings prompt relief but aggravates the condition. A person who drinks enough alcohol to keep his blood sugar up soon becomes very drunk as well as malnourished.

The hypoglycemia and malnutrition of alcoholic patients should be treated promptly. Large doses of Vitamins B1 (Thiamin), B6 (Pyridoxine), and Niacinamide are especially useful for controlling alcohol withdrawal symptoms and correcting the hypoglycemic metabolism. These vitamins, along with generous amounts of other vitamins and a high protein, low carbohydrate diet, should be continued indefinitely to reduce the craving for alcohol.

Acupuncture is not a substitute for a good diet but can be used to relieve withdrawal symptoms, regulate metabolism, and give the patient a feeling of well-being which makes it easier for him to give up alcohol. Acupuncture treatments should be given once or twice a day until ten treatments have been given. Many of our patients have remained free from alcohol for over three years after one such course of treatment. Others have returned for another series of treatments after several months of abstinence. A few have found that acupuncture once a week or once a month was needed for maintenance of their sobriety.

The acupuncture points most frequently used for treating withdrawal symptoms are:

Meridian points: St 8 · Br 20 · GB 20 and 34 · UB 10 and 54 · Co 4 and 11 · Lu 7 · Sp 1 and 6 · Ki 1

Auricular points: Brain · Liver · Kidney · Spleen · Stomach

Other points used in subsequent treatments for alcoholism are:

Meridian points: Co 10 and 15 · Br 26 · Va 7 · He 7 · Sx 4 and 12 · SI 3 · UB 11, 15, and 60 · St 25, 40, and 44 · Me 6

These points should be used bilaterally in most cases and can be used along with points for treating the patient's other medical problems. It is, of course, not necessary or desirable to use all these points for every treatment.

All alcoholics should be given psychotherapy as well as diet therapy along with acupuncture. Conjoint therapy with their spouses or family may be especially helpful because most of them have domestic problems which may trigger episodes of heavy drinking. They should be encouraged to attend Alcoholics Anonymous meetings and reminded that excessive coffee drinking has an adverse effect on the hypoglycemia which is often associated with alcoholism.

Smoking Addiction

Although it is generally agreed that smoking is a health hazard, many people enjoy it and seem unable to discontinue this habit without help. Acupuncture may help people increase their will power enough to stop smoking. It relieves the withdrawal symptoms of nervousness, insomnia, depression, and craving for excessive amounts of food. Most people experience a feeling of well-being and self-confidence after acupuncture treatment.

Inserting a staple in the ear and leaving it there for weeks is an American innovation which is seldom effective. It also promotes infection and keloid formation. Regular acupuncture treatments are more effective and safer. Most people are able to stop smoking after their first treatment but should have six for continuing relief from smoking addiction.

Nutritional therapy should be started along with acupuncture to help the body recover from the effects of smoking. Vitamin A (20,000 units); Vitamin C (3 gm.); Vitamin E (400 units); Niacinamide (500 mg.); Pantothenate (300 mg.); Thiamin, Riboflavin, and Pyridoxine (50 mg. each); and B12 (500 mcg.) daily are usually prescribed.

Acupuncture points include:

Meridian points: Lu 4 and 7 · Co 4 and 13 · St 36 and 40 · Sp 8 · Br 24 · He 7 · Va 6

Auricular points: Shenmen · Lung · Abdomen · Pharynx · Internal Nose · Kidney · Maxillary Sinus

Obesity

Inserting acupuncture needles superficially into various parts of the body can facilitate weight loss by giving the person a feeling of well-being which can suppress the desire for excessive food. Acupuncture can also stimulate metabolism and thereby enable the body to utilize food efficiently instead of storing it as fat.

The specific points used for each patient at each treatment depend on many individual factors. The same points are not used for everybody, and the same points are not even used for the same patient at each treatment. Both the physician who examines the patient before treatment and the acupuncturist determine which points should be used with regard to the patient's fat distribution, emotional status, eating habits, and other factors.

The use of staples in the ear for weight control is an American innovation which is often ineffective and dangerous. Only two points—one in each ear—are used by this method in contrast to the ten or twenty points used in regular acupuncture treatments. The cartilage of the ear does not replace itself after injury and has little resistance to infection. Staples left in place for many days promote infection and sometimes fall out and enter the ear canal, where they can damage the eardrum or other structures. There have been cases of people having permanent holes in the upper parts of their ears as the result of infected staples with sloughing. For these reasons, we do not recommend the use of ear staples for weight reduction.

Diet and exercise are helpful in any program of weight reduction. Each patient should discuss his diet and exercise habits with the physician who examines him. Most people who come for acupuncture treatments, however, have been given diets and exercise regimens before. They may have good knowledge of what they should and shouldn't eat, but they feel depressed or irritable when they try to stay on a diet. Acupuncture should relieve such problems and improve willpower.

The weight loss to be expected is about two to four pounds a week. Six to ten acupuncture treatments are usually sufficient, and these can be given once or twice a week. Weight loss should continue after the treatments are completed until normal weight is achieved. The effects of acupuncture usually last at least six months and sometimes a year or more. If the desire to eat excessively returns at any time in the future, a few more acupuncture treatments should relieve it.

Acupuncture points for weight control include:

Meridian points: St 25 and 36 · Sp 6 and 9 · Me 6 · Sx 4, 6, 8, and 11 · Va 6 and 9

Auricular points: Lung · Liver · Kidney · Brain · Small Intestine · Colon

The needles are usually inserted bilaterally. The selection of points to use for each treatment depends on the evaluation of the patient's condition and response to previous treatment.

AUTISTIC DISORDERS

Autism is self-centeredness so severe that it causes inability to relate to other people. The autistic person is preoccupied with his own body and mind to the extent that he is oblivious to the world around him and unable to recognize that other people are similar to him and have feelings as real as his own. He treats people as if they are things and ignores what they say and do unless their actions restrict his movement or cause him pain.

Emotional development begins in infancy and continues throughout life. All babies are born "autistic" but normally begin to respond to other people by smiling and trying to communicate with them in other ways before they are six months old. Failure of emotional development is often related to deprivation of affection. Severe psychological trauma may cause arrest of emotional development at any stage from infancy on. The severity of autism is usually related to how early emotional development was arrested.

In a broad sense, emotional development may be measured by the degree to which a person is able to empathize and communicate with other people. Severe psychological trauma or prolonged frustration frequently produces emotional regression and increased self-centeredness. Depression, anxiety, and neurotic or psychotic behavior are evidence of self–preoccupation. The severity of the symptoms is related to the extent of self–preoccupation.

Psychotherapy may be aimed at identifying the psychological trauma and emotional education or reeducation to increase the patient's ability to empathize and communicate with other people.

Acupuncture is not a substitute for psychotherapy, but it is usually more effective than psychotropic drugs in giving a patient relief from emotional pain along with feelings of well-being that make him receptive to psychotherapy or willing and able to work out solutions to his emotional problems without professional help.

There is increasing evidence that metabolic abnormalities are associated with autistic disorders and that correcting these may relieve symptoms considerably. Whether these result from emotional trauma or whether these are congenital and predispose to self-sensitivity and autism is not yet clear. In any case, nutritional therapy should be given along with acupuncture and continued afterward to minimize metabolic problems.

Childhood Autism

Autism is deficiency of response to other people. Autistic children do not imitate people and learn to speak like other children, although they may have normal or high intelligence. This autistic behavior pattern becomes evident in the preschool years and may cause children to be considered mentally retarded because they ignore most attempts to communicate with them. They seem to be more interested in things than in people but may be very responsive to music.

The cause of autism has not been determined, but there is considerable evidence that it is related to metabolic abnormalities, allergic reactions, or nutritional deficiencies. Various types of psychotherapy, however, have been more successful than medication as treatment. Although sedatives or stimulants may cause a temporary change in behavior, they have serious side effects and may cause addiction.

According to acupuncture theory, autism is due to imbalances in the body energy system which can be corrected by acupuncture treatments. Acupuncture can regulate metabolism and reduce allergic responses. The Washington Acupuncture Center has treated more than 100 autistic children successfully. Most autistic children show significant improvement in responsiveness by the time they have had six treatments, but many more are usually required to enable the child to function normally.

Psychotherapy and nutritional therapy can be given along with acupuncture and should be continued afterwards. The autistic child should have a diet free from anything to which he is known to be allergic, artificial food dyes, preservatives, and other toxic substances. All drugs should be discontinued, but such drugs as amphetamines, barbiturates, Valium, and cortisone derivatives must be discontinued gradually to avoid serious withdrawal reactions.

Although children may not cooperate well with acupuncture therapy at first, they usually become surprisingly willing to have the needles inserted as they begin to improve after the first few treatments. Apparently they soon discover that the treatments are not very painful and are helping them to function better.

Classical points most frequently used are:

Meridian points: Lu 9 · Co 4 and 11 · Sp 6 and 10 · UB 1, 12, and 54 · GB 20 · Ki 6 · Va 5, 7, and 9 · Me 5 and 17 · Sx 23

Auricular points: Brain · Liver · Kidney · Stomach · Sympathy

Schizophrenia

Schizophrenia is a mental and emotional disorder characterized by autism, delusional thinking, irrational behavior, inappropriate emotions, withdrawal from reality, and sometimes auditory hallucinations. The person with this behavior pattern is so preoccupied with his own body and his own thoughts that he becomes less and less concerned with other people and his environment. It has been called the "whirlpool of self-centeredness." The onset of this condition is usually between the ages of 12 and 50.

Although many psychiatrists, especially psychoanalysts, still insist that there is no physiologic basis for schizophrenia, recent biochemical research has demonstrated metabolic abnormalities. Physical abnormalities, such as brain tumors and some diseases, also can produce schizophrenic symptoms.

Some drugs, such as cortisone, can promote the development of schizophrenia. Tranquilizing drugs, such as Thorazine, can relieve the symptoms temporarily and make patients more comfortable and cooperative, but they damage the basal ganglia of the brain and may produce dyskinesia and other serious side effects.

Acupuncture is a safe and effective treatment for schizophrenia. In most cases, it can replace dangerous drugs. It can be given along with psychotherapy and nutritional therapy.

Patients recovering from schizophrenia should take Vitamin C (3 gm.), B1 (20 mg.), B6 (20 mg.), Niacinamide (1 gm.), Pantothenic acid (200 mg.), Biotin (20 mcg.), calcium (1 gm.), zinc (30 mg.), and other essential nutrients daily for the rest of their lives. They should avoid food with artificial preservatives and dyes.

Acupuncture points for treating schizophrenia include:

Meridian points: St 36 and 40 · GB 2 and 20 · Me 5 and 17 · UB 1 · Va 5 and 7 · Li 2 and 3 · Sx 23 · Br 13, 14, 15, and 26 · SI 19 · Co 4 and 11 · Sp 6 and 10 · Lu 9 · Ki 6

Auricular points: Brain · Liver · Kidney · Stomach · Sympathy

LIST OF ACUPUNCTURE POINTS ON THE MAJOR MERIDIANS

Lung = Lu = A = Shou Tai Yin Fei Ching, Hand-Taiyin

1, Chungfu, Zhongfu
2, Yunmen
3, Tienfu, Tianfu
4, Hsiapai, Xaibai
5, Chihtse, Chize
6, Kungtsui, Kongzui
7, Liehchueh, Lieque

8, Chingchu, Jingqu

9, Taiyuan

10, Yuchi, Yuji

11, Shaoshang

Colon = Co = B = Large Intestine = Shou Yang Min Ta Chang Ching, Hand-Yangming

1, Shangyang

2, Erhchien, Erjian

3, Sanchien, Sanjian

4, Hoko, Hegu

5, Yangshi, Yangxi

6, Pienli, Pianli

7, Wenliu

8, Hsialien, Xialian

9, Shanglien, Shanglian

10, Shousanli

11, Chuchih, Quchi

12, Chouliao, Zhouliao

13, Shouwuli, Wuli

14, Pinao, Binao

15, Chienyu, Jianyu

16, Chuku, Jugu

17, Tienting, Tianding

18, Futu, Neck-Futu

19, Holiao, Nose-Heliao

20, Yinghsiang, Yingxiang

Stomach = St = C Tsu Yang Ming Wei Ching, Foot-Yangming

1, Chengchi, Chengqi

2, Szupai, Sibai

3, Chuliao, Juliao

4, Titsang, Dicang

5, Taying, Daying

6,   Chiache, Jiache

7,   Hsiakuan, Xiaguan

8,   Touwei

9,   Jenying, Renying

10,   Shuitu

11,   Chishe, Qishi

12,   Chuehpen, Quepen

13,   Chihu, Qihu

14,   Kufang

15,   Wuyi

16,   Yinchuang, Yingchuang

17,   Juchung, Ruzhong

18,   Juken, Rugen

19,   Puyung, Burong

20,   Chengman

21,   Liangmen

22,   Kuanmen, Guanmen

23,   Taiyi

24,   Huajoumen, Huaroumen

25,   Tienshu, Tianshu

26,   Wailing

27,   Tachu, Daju

28,   Shuitao, Shuidao

29,   Kueilai, Guilai

30,   Chichung, Qichong

31,   Pikuan, Biguan

32,   Futu

33,   Yinshih, Yinshi

34,   Liangchiu, Liangqiu

35,   Tupi, Dubi

36,   Tsusanli, Zusanli

37,   Shangchushu, Shangjuxu

38,   Tiaoku, Tiaokou

39,   Hsiachushu, Xiajuxu

40, Fenglung, Fenglong

41, Chiehhsi, Jiexi

42, Chungyang, Chongyang

43, Hsienku, Xiangu

44, Neitieng, Neiting

45, Litui, Lidui

Spleen = Sp = D = Tsu Tai Yin Pi Ching, Foot-Taiyin

1, Yinpai, Yinbai

2, Tatu, Dadu

3, Taipai, Taibai

4, Kungsun, Gongsun

5, Shangchiu, Shangqiu

6, Shanyinchiao, Shanyinjiao

7, Louku, Lougu

8, Tichi, Diji

9, Yinlinchuan, Yinlingquan

10, Hsiehhai, Xuehai

11, Chimen, Jimen

12, Chungmen, Chongmen

13, Fushe

14, Fuchieh, Fujie

15, Taheng, Daheng

16, Fuai

17, Shihtou, Shidou

18, Tienhsi, Tianxi

19, Hsiunghsiang, Xiongxiang

20, Chouyung, Zourong

21, Tapao, Tabao

Heart = He = E = Shou Shao Yin Hsin Ching, Hand-Shaoyin

1, Chichuan, Jiquan

2, Chingling, Qingling

3, Shaohai

4,   Lingtao, Lingdao

5,   Tungli, Tongli

6,   Yinhsi, Yinxi

7,   Shenmen

8,   Shaofu

9,   Shaochung, Shaochong

Small Intestine = SI = F = Shou Tai Yang Hsiao Chang Ching, Hand-Taiyang

1,   Shaotse, Shaoze

2,   Chienku, Qiangu

3,   Houshsi, Houxi

4,   Wanku, Wangu

5,   Yangku, Yanggu

6,   Yanglao, Zhizheng

7,   Chihcheng, Zhizheng

8,   Hsiaohai, Xiaohai

9,   Chienchen, Jianzhen

10, Naoshu

11, Tientsung, Tianzong

12, Pingfeng, Bingfeng

13, Chuyuan, Quyuan

14, Chienwaishu, Jianwaishu

15, Chienchungshu, Jianzhongshu

16, Tienchuang, Tianchuang

17, Tienjung, Tianrong

18, Chuanliao, Quanliao

19, Tingkung, Tinggong

Urinary Bladder = UB = G = Tsu Tai Yang Pang Kuang Ching, Foot-Taiyang

1,   Chingming, Jingming

2,   Tsanchu, Zanzhu

3,   Meichung, Meichong

4,   Chucha, Quchai

5,   Wuchu

6,   Chengkung, Chengguang

7,   Tungtien, Tongtian

8,   Lochueh, Luoque

9,   Yuchen, Yuzhen

10,   Tienchu, Tianzhu

11,   Tachu, Dashu

12,   Fengmen

13,   Feishu

14,   Chuehyinshu, Jueyyinshu

15,   Hsinshu, Xinshu

16,   Tushu, Dushu

17,   Keshu, Geshu

18,   Kanshu, Ganshu

19,   Tanshu, Danshu

20,   Pishu

21,   Weishu

22,   Sanchiaoshu, Sanjiaoshu

23,   Shenshu

24,   Chihaishu, Qihaishu

25,   Tachangshu, Dachangshu

26,   Kuanguanshu, Quanyuanshu

27,   Hsiaochangshu, Xiaochangshu

28,   Pankuangshu, Pangguangshu

29,   Chunglushu, Zhonglushu

30,   Paihuanshu, Baihuanshu

31,   Shangliao

32,   Tzuliao

33,   Chungliao, Zhongliao

34,   Hsialiao, Xialiao

35,   Huiyang

36,   Fufen, Changfu

37,   Pohu, Yinmen

38,   Kaohuang, Fuxi

39,   Shentang, Weiyang

40,   Yihsi, Weizhong

41,   Kekuan, Fufen

42,   Hunmen, Pohu

43,   Yangkang, Gaohuang

44,   Yishe, Shentang

45,   Weitsang, Yixi

46,   Huangmen, Geguan

47,   Chihshih, Hunmen

48,   Paohuang, Yanggang

49,   Chihpien, Yishi

50,   Chengfu, Weicang

51,   Yenmen, Huangmen

52,   Fuhsi, Zhishi

53,   Weiyang, Baohuang

54,   Weichung, Zhibian

55,   Heyang

56,   Chengchin, Chengjin

57,   Chengshan

58,   Feiyang

59,   Fuyang

60,   Kunlun

61,   Pushen

62,   Shenmo, Shenmai

63,   Chimen, Jinmen

64,   Chingku, Jinggu

65,   Shuku, Shugu

66,   Tungku, Tonggu

67,   Chihyin, Zhiyin

Kidney = Ki = H = Tsu Shao Yin Sheng Ching, Foot-Shaoyin

1,   Yungchuan, Yongquan

2,   Janku, Rangu

3,   Taihsi, Taixi

4,   Tachung, Dazhong

5,   Shuichuan, Shuiquan

6,   Chaohai, Zhaohai

7,   Fuliu

8,   Chiaohsin, Jiaoxin

9,   Chupin, Zhubin

10,   Yinku, Yingu

11,   Hengku, Henggu

12,   Taheh, Dahe

13,   Chihsueh, Qixue

14,   Szuman, Siman

15,   Chungchu, Zhongzhu

16,   Huangshu

17,   Shangchu, Shangqu

18,   Shihkuan, Shiguan

19,   Yintu, Yindu

20,   Tungku, Tonggu

21,   Yumen, Youmen

22,   Pulang, Bulang

23,   Shenfeng

24,   Linghsu, Lingxu

25,   Shentsang, Shencang

26,   Yuchung, Yuzhong

27,   Shufu

Vascular = Va = Pericardium = I = Heart Governor = Circulation = Shou Chueh Yin Hsin Pao Ching, Hand-Jueyin

1,   Tienchih, Tianchi

2,   Tienchuan, Tianquan

3,   Chutse, Quze

4,   Hsimen, Ximen

5,   Chienshih, Jianshi

6,   Neikuan, Neiguan

7, Taling, Daling

8, Laokung, Laogong

9, Chungchung, Zhongchong

Metabolism = Me = J = Triple Warmer = Shou Shao Yang San Chiao Ching, Sanjiao, Hand-Shaoyang

1, Kuanchung, Guanchong

2, Yemen

3, Chungchu, Zhongzhu

4, Yangchih, Yangchi

5, Waikuan, Waiguan

6, Chihkou, Zhigou

7, Huitsung, Huizong

8, Sanyanglo, Sanyangluo

9, Szutu, Sidu

10, Tienching, Tianjing

11, Chinglengyuan, Qinglengyuan

12, Hiaolo, Xiaoluo

13, Naohui

14, Chienliao, Jianliao

15, Tienliao, Tianliao

16, Tienyu, Tianyou

17, Yifeng

18, Chihmo, Qimai

19, Luhsi, Luxi

20, Chuehsun, Jiaosun

21, *Erhem, Ermen*

22, Ear-*Heliao*

23, *Szuchukung, Sizhukong*

Gall Bladder = GB = K = Tsu Shao Yang Tan Ching, Foot-Shaoyang

1, Tungtsuliao, Tongziliao

2, Tinghui

3, Shangkuan, Shanguan

4,   Hanyen, Hanyan

5,   Hsuanlu, Xuanlu

6,   Hsuanli, Xuanli

7,   Chupin, Qubin

8,   Shuaiku, Shuaigu

9,   Tienchung, Tianchong

10, Fupai, Fubai

11, Chiaoyin, Qiaoyin

12, Wanku, Wangu

13, Penshen, Benshen

14, Yangpai, Yangbai

15, Linchi, Linqi

16, Muchuang

17, Chengying, Zhengying

18, Chengling

19, Naokung, Naokong

20, Fengchih, Fangchi

21, Chienchin, Jianjing

22, Yuanyeh, Yuanye

23, Chechin, Zhejin

24, Jihyueh, Riyue

25, Chingmen, Jingmen

26, Taimo, Daimai

27, Wushu

28, Weitao, Weidao

29, Chuliao, Juliao

30, Huantiao

31, Fengshih, Fengshi

32, Chungtu, Zhongdu

33, Yangkuan, Xiyangguan

34, Yanglinchuan, Yanglingquan

35, Yangchiao, Yangjiao

36, Waichiu, Waiqiu

37, Kuangming, Guangming
38, Yangfu
39, Hsuanchung, Xuanzhong
40, Chiuhsu, Qiuxu
41, Linchi, Linqi
42, Tiwuhui, Diwuhui
43, Hsiahsi, Xiaxi
44, Chiaoyin, Qiaoyin

Liver = Li = L = Tsu Chueh Yin Kan Ching, Foot-Jueyin

1, Tatun, Dadun
2, Hsingchien, Xingjian
3, Taichung, Taichong
4, Chungfeng, Zhongfeng
5, Likou, Ligou
6, Chungtu, Zhongdu
7, Hsikuan, Xiguan
8, Chuchuan, Ququan
9, Yinpao, Yinbao
10, Wuli
11, Yinlien, Yinlian
12, Chimo, Jimai
13, Changman, Zhangmen
14, Chimen, Qimen

Sex = Sx = M = Conception Vessel = Jen Mo = Ren Mo

1, Huiyin
2, Chuku, Qugu
3, Chungchi, Zhongji
4, Kuanyuan, Quanyuan
5, Shihmen
6, Chihai, Qihai
7, Yinchiao, Yinjiao

8,   Chinchung, or Shenjue

9,   Shuifen

10,   Hsiawan, Xiawan

11,   Chienli, Jianli

12,   Chungwan, Zhongwan

13,   Shangwan

14,   Chuchueh, Jujue

15,   Chiuwei, Jiuwei

16,   Chungting, Zhongting

17,   Shanchung, Shanzhong

18,   Yutang

19,   Tzukai, Zigong

20,   Huakai, Huangai

21,   Hsuanchi, Xuanji

22,   Tientu, Tiantu

23,   Lienchuan, Lianquan

24,   Chengchiang, Chengjiang

Brain = Br = N = Governor Vessel = Tu Mo = Du Mo

1,   Changchiang, Changqiang

2,   Yaoshu

3,   Yangkuan, Yaoyangguan

4,   Mingmen

5,   Hsuanshu, Xuanshu

6,   Chichung, Jizhong

7,   Chungshu, Zhongshu

8,   Chinso, Jinsuo

9,   Chihyang, Zhiyang

10,   Lingtai

11,   Shentao, Shendao

12,   Shenchu, Shenzhu

13,   Taotao, Taodao

14,   Tachui, Dazhui

15,   Yamen

16,   Fengfu
17,   Naohu
18,   Chiangchien, Qiangjian
19,   Houting, Houding
20,   Paihui, Baihui
21,   Chienting, Qianding
22,   Hsinhui, Xinhui
23,   Shanghsing, Shangxing
24,   Shenting
25,   Suliao
26,   Jenchung, Renzhong
27,   Tuituan, Duiduan
28,   Yinchiao, Yinjiao

SPECIFIC POINTS
FOR VARIOUS
CONDITIONS

SPECIFIC POINTS FOR VARIOUS CONDITIONS

Medical Conditions	Points on Major Meridians	Auricular Points
Analgesia		
Intracranial	Co 4 • Va 6 • SI 18 • St 43 • Li 3 • UB 2 • GB 2, 8 and 41 • Br 20 • Me 21	Shenmen • Sympathy • Forehead • Lung • Kidney
Eyes	Co 4 • St 1, 2, and 7 • Me 5 • Va 6 • UB 2 • SI 6 • GB 4 and 37 • Li 3	Eye • Eye I • Eye II • Forehead • Lung • Liver • Kidney • Shenmen • Sympathy
Ears	Co 4 • Me 3 and 17 • Va 6 • St 2, 3, and 44	
Nose	Co 4 and 20 • St 2 and 3 • Va 6 • SI 3	Forehead • Internal Nose • External Nose • Lung • Shenmen • Sympathy
Maxilla	Co 4, 11, and 20 • St 2 and 3 • Me 5 and 6 • Va 6 • St 36	Maxilla • Forehead • External Nose • Internal Nose • Kidney • Shenmen • Sympathy
Larynx	Co 4 • Me 6 • St 44	Larynx • Pharynx • Neck • Lung • Kidney • Shenmen • Sympathy
Tonsillectomy	Co 4 • Me 6 • Li 3 • Ki 7 • Va 6 • St 44	Pharynx • Larynx • Tonsil
Mandible	Co 4 • St 40 and 43 • GB 38 and 43 • UB 60 • Li 3 • Sp 4 • Va 6	
Cleft Palate Surgery	Co 4 and 20 • Va 4 and 6 • GB 38 • St 6, 7, and 40 • Br 26 • Sx 24 • SI 18	
Upper Teeth	Co 4 • St 6, 7, and 44	
Lower Teeth	Co 4 • St 5 and 6	
Esophagus	Co 4 • Va 6 • St 6 • GB 31	
Neck, including Thyroid	Co 4 and 18 • Va 6 • St 6 and 44 • GB 31	Shenmen • Lung • Neck • Pharynx • Larynx

Surgery	Body Points	Ear Points
Chest Surgery	Co 4 and 14 • Va 4 and 6 • Me 5, 6, 8, and 14 • Br 11 and 14	Shenmen • Lung • Kidney • Thoracic • Heart • Esophagus • Sympathy
Stomach and Intestines	St 36 and 37 • Me 17 • Va 6	Shenmen • Abdomen • Colon • Stomach • Lung • Diaphragm • Small Intestine • Sympathy
Gall Bladder and Biliary Duct Surgery	St 36 • Sp 6	Gall Bladder • Liver • Stomach • Lung • Diaphragm • Pancreas • Abdomen • Shenmen • Sympathy
Splenectomy	St 36 • Sp 4 and 6 • Li 3 and 13 • Sx 15 • Va 4 • Co 4	Spleen • Abdomen • Lung • Shenmen • Sympathy
Appendectomy	St 36 • GB 20	Appendix • Abdomen • Lung • Colon • Small Intestine • Sympathy • Shenmen
Herniorrhaphy	St 36 • GB 28 • UB 18 and 25 • Sp 15	Abdomen • Sympathy • Knee
Gynecological and Obstetrical Surgery	St 36 • Li 6 • GB 26 and 34 • Sp 6 and 9 • Br 2 and 4 • UB 32 and 33 • Sx 4 • Li 3	Shenmen • Sympathy • Uterus • Gonads • Lung • Abdomen • Kidney
Urological Surgery	Br 2 • St 36 and 43 • GB 27, 28, and 38 • UB 34 and 60 • Ki 3 • Li 3 and 5 • Sp 3 and 6 • Co 4 • Me 5 • SI 3 • Va 4 • Sx 3 and 4	Shenmen • Sympathy • Lung • Kidney • Abdomen • Urinary Bladder
Hemorrhoidectomy	UB 30 and 39	Rectum • Lung • Sympathy • Shenmen
Shoulder and Elbow Surgery or Manipulation	Va 4 and 6 • Co 4, 15, and 18 • Me 5	Shenmen • Sympathy • Shoulder • Lung • Kidney • Elbow
Arm and Hand Surgery	Co 4, 11, and 15 • He 2 and 3 • Lu 2, 5, and 10 • GB 34 • UB 54 • St 36	Shenmen • Sympathy • Lung • Shoulder • Elbow • Kidney
Hip and Leg Surgery	St 31, 36, 40, and 44 • UB 40, 59, and 60 • GB 30, 31, 34, 39, and 43 • Li 3 and 5 • Sp 6, 9, 10, and 12 • Ki 3	Shenmen • Sympathy • Lung • Knee • Hip • Buttocks • Kidney • Toes • Ankle

SPECIFIC POINTS FOR VARIOUS CONDITIONS (Continued)

Medical Conditions	Points on Major Meridians	Auricular Points
Lumbar Laminectomy	Co 4 • Me 5 • Va 6 • Br 3 and 4	Shenmen • Sympathy • Lung • Kidney • Lumbar
Allergies, General	Br 10 and 14 • UB 10, 11, 13, 14, 25, 26, 38, 54, and 57 • Sx 6, 12, 14, 17, and 22 • Lu 1 and 7 • St 25, 36, and 40 • Co 4 and 11 • GB 20 and 30 • SI 14 • Li 10 • Va 6 • Me 5 • Ki 3 • Sp 6	Lung • Internal Nose • Maxillary Sinus • Stomach • Small Intestine • Liver
Asthma, Acute attack	St 3–6 • Me 3–6 • UB 12 and 13 • Lu 5 • Sx 17	Lung • Shenmen • Sympathy
Asthma, Chronic	UB 12, 23, and 38 • Sx 6, 12, 14, and 22 • Lu 7 • Br 14 • Co 4 • GB 20	Lung • Internal Nose • Maxillary Sinus
Hay Fever	Co 4, 19, and 20 • Lu 1 and 9 • GB 20 • SI 36 • St 18 • Br 16, 20 and 23	Lung • Internal Nose • Maxillary Sinus
Rhinitis, Chronic	Co 4, 11, 19, and 20 • GB 20 • Br 16, 20, and 23 • Sp 6 • SI 36	Internal Nose • Maxillary Sinus
Sinusitis, Chronic	Lu 9 • Co 4, 19, and 20 • SI 2 and 36 • GB 20 • Me 22 • UB 10 • St 36 • Br 14, 16, 20 and 23	Internal Nose • Maxillary Sinus • Liver
Circulatory Disorders		
Hypertension	SI 14 • UB 11 • GB 20 and 21 • Li 13 and 14 • Sx 5 and 15	Kidney • Genitalia • Gonads • Liver • Sympathy
Edema	Lu 7 • Co 4 and 6 • Sp 6 and 9 • UB 20, 23, 28, and 39 • Br 4 • St 36	Kidney • Heart • Liver • Abdomen • Urinary Bladder • Shenmen
Angina Pectoris	Me 4 and 6 • Co 4 and 11 • Sp 17 • St 3, 6, and 36 • Br 14 and 20 • UB 13, 20, and 24 • Lu, 1 and 7 • Sx 9, 12, 17, and 22 • Va 6 • Li 3 and 10 • Ki 6 and 7 • GB 20	Lung • Heart • Liver • Gall Bladder • Pancreas • Sympathy
Buerger's Disease	St 25, 29, and 30 • Sp 14 and 15 • GB 26 • Va 4 and 5 • Me 5–7 • Sx 5 and 6	Ankle • Toes • Knee • Gall Bladder • Colon • Liver • Sympathy • Shenmen

304

Raynaud's Syndrome	Co 3, 4, and 11 • He 4 and 7 • Lu 3 and 8 • St 36 and 39 • GB 33 • Sp 6	Fingers • Toes • Ankle • Sympathy • Shenmen
Dermatologic Disorders, General	Lu 3 and 5 • Co 4, 11, and 16 • St 36 • Sp 10 and 20 • UB 12, 13, 54, and 57 • Ki 26 • GB 30, 31, 35, 38, and 39 • Br 14	Liver • Kidney • Colon • Small Intestine
Eczema	Co 11 • Sp 10 • UB 12, 13, 54, and 57 • GB 20, 30, 31, 38, and 39 • Br 14	Abdomen • Knee • Elbow • Sympathy
Acne Rosacea	UB 1 and 40 • Sp 6 and 10 • Co 4 and 11 • St 1 • Lu 7 • GB 20 and 37	Liver • Kidney
Acne Vulgaris	Lu 3 and 5 • Co 4, 11, and 16 • Sp 20 • Ki 26 • St 36 • GB 35	Gonads • Liver • External Nose • Spleen • Stomach • Shenmen
Psoriasis	Co 4, 11, and 15 • St 36 • Sp 6 and 10 • UB 6, 12, 54, and 60 • Va 3 • GB 20, 30, 31, 38, and 39 • Br 20	Liver • Kidney • Knee • Elbow • Ankle • Spleen • Buttocks • Shenmen
Pruritus (Itching)	Co 11 • Sp 10 • UB 12, 13, 54, and 57 • GB 20 • Br 14 and 20	Liver • Kidney • Shenmen
Alopecia (Baldness)	Br 14 • Co 11 • Va 6 • Ki 1 and 3 • UB 23 and 40 • Li 2, 13, and 14 • GB 20 • Sp 10	Liver • Gonads • Pancreas • Kidney
Hyperhidrosis	Co 4 and 11 • Ki 7 • St 36 • Sp 4 • GB 21 • Li 3 • Sx 6 • Br 14 and 20	Kidney • Liver • Forehead • Brain • Pancreas
Wrinkles	St 2, 4, 6, and 37 • Sp 4 • He 7 • Ki 1 and 3 • Li 2 • Sx 24 • Br 16 and 25	Eye I • Eye II • Gonads • Liver • Kidney • Neck • Forehead • External Nose • Stomach • Genitalia • Colon
Gastro-intestinal Disorders		
Peptic Ulcer Disease	St 36, 37, and 44 • UB 10, 11, 17, 18, 21, and 22 • GB 20 • Sp 4	Stomach • Small Intestine • Liver • Pancreas

SPECIFIC POINTS FOR VARIOUS CONDITIONS (Continued)

Medical Conditions	Points on Major Meridians	Auricular Points
Abdominal Pain, Post-operative	Co 4 • St 25, 36, and 40 • Va 6 • UB 25 • Me 6 • Li 3 • Sx 6 and 14	Stomach • Small Intestine • Liver • Pancreas • Colon • Shenmen
Abdominal Pain, Chronic	Co 4 and 11 • UB 18 • St 36 • Va 6 • Li 3 • Sp 4 • He 7	Same as Post-operative
Colitis	Co 3 and 4 • St 25, 36, 37 and 44 • Sp 3, 4, 6, and 15 • UB 17–19, 21–23, and 25 • Li 2, 3, and 12 • Sx 6, 10, 12, 13, 14, and 17 • GB 20 • Va 6	Pancreas • Abdomen • Colon • Small Intestine • Shenmen • Liver • Kidney
Constipation	Co 7 • St 25 and 40 • Sp 3 and 15 • UB 25 • Ki 3 • Me 6 • Sx 6	Sympathy • Pancreas • Colon • Rectum • Liver • Small Intestine • Stomach • Abdomen
Hiatus Hernia	Co 11 and 15 • St 25, 26, and 40 • UB 23, 25, and 54 • GB 30 • Me 6 • Li 3 • Sx 6 and 14	Diaphragm • Abdomen • Stomach • Esophagus • Shenmen • Sympathy
Hiccups	UB 17–19, and 21 • Sx 12 and 22 • Va 6 • SI 14 • GB 24 and 40 • Li 13 • Me 6 • St 25 • Sp 6	Diaphragm • Esophagus • Stomach • Abdomen • Neck • Shenmen • Sympathy
Ileus	Co 4 • St 25, 36, and 40 • UB 25 • Me 6 • Li 3 • Sx 6 and 14	Small Intestine • Stomach • Colon • Abdomen • Liver • Pancreas
Indigestion	Co 3 and 4 • St 36 • Sp 4 and 5 • UB 17–19 • GB 20 • Va 6 • Sx 14 and 17	Stomach • Abdomen • Small Intestine • Liver • Pancreas • Colon • Diaphragm
Vomiting	St 36 • Va 6 • St 25 and 40 • Me 6 • Li 3	Esophagus • Stomach • Small Intestine • Liver • Diaphragm • Shenmen • Sympathy
Genital Disorders		
Sexual Dysfunction	St 36 • Sp 6 and 9 • UB 23, 32, and 52 • GB 3 • Sx 3 and 4 • Li 8 • Br 4	Gonads • Urethra • Genitalia • Lumbar • Brain
Amenorrhea	Co 4, 15, and 18 • St 25 and 36 • Sx 3 and 4 • Sp 6, 8, and 10 • Va 6 • Br 14 • UB 11, 18, 21, 31–33 • Li 8 • GB 20 • He 6 and 7 • Me 6 and 8 • Lu 2, 5, and 10 • SI 3	Gonads • Uterus • Liver • Spleen • Genitalia

Breast Hypoplasia	Sx 17 • St 19 • He 2 • SI 4 • Co 11	Gonads • Uterus • Liver • Brain
Penis Hypoplasia	Lu 3, 4, and 10 • He 4, 6, and 8 • Va 4 and 8 • Sp 3 and 6 • St 36 and 44 • GB 34 and 43 • Sx 5 and 7 • Br 24	Genitalia • Gonads • Buttocks • Brain • Sympathy • Liver
Infertility	St 33 • Sp 4 and 8 • UB 23 and 25 • Li 3 and 8 • Sx 2–6 • Br 4	Gonads • Uterus • Lumbar • Liver • Brain
Menstrual Disorders	Co 4, 15, and 18 • St 25 and 36 • Sp 6, 8, and 10 • UB 11, 18, 21, 31, 32, and 33 • He 6 and 7 • Me 6 and 8 • Lu 2, 5, and 10 • GB 20 • SI 3 • Sx 3 and 4 • Br 14	Genitalia • Uterus • Urinary Bladder • Abdomen • Shenmen • Sympathy
Obstetrics Induction of Labor	See Obstetrical Analgesia Co 4 • St 36 • Sp 6	
Menopausal Syndrome	Co 11 • St 19, 29, and 30 • Sp 6 and 8 • UB 23 and 25 • SI 1 • He 2 • Li 3 and 8 • Sx 4 and 17	Liver • Kidney • Uterus • Gonads • Genitalia • Brain

Musculoskeletal Disorders

Arthritis, General	Co 4, 10, 11, and 15 • St 36 • Sp 4 • Me 6 • GB 20, 21, 30, 34, and 39 • Br 14	Sympathy • Shenmen • Liver • Kidney • Brain
Cervical	Co 11, 15, and 16 • SI 19 • GB 14	Neck • Shoulder
Spinal	UB 10–35, and 38 • Br 4, 11, and 14	Neck • Thoracic • Lumbar • Sacral
Elbows	Co 11 • St 36 • GB 21	Elbow
Wrists and Hands	Me 4–6 • Co 5, 6, and 11 • SI 4 and 7 • He 7 • Va 5 and 7 • Sp 10	Fingers
Thumbs	Co 4–6 • Lu 9–11	Fingers
Index Fingers	Co 1–3 • Va 7 and 8	Fingers
Middle Fingers	Va 9 • Me 3	Fingers

SPECIFIC POINTS FOR VARIOUS CONDITIONS (Continued)

Medical Conditions	Points on Major Meridians	Auricular Points
Ring Fingers	Me 1–3 • He 8 • SI 5	Fingers
Little Fingers	SI 2 and 3 • He 7 and 8	Fingers
Hips	GB 30, 31, and 34 • UB 30, 31, 48, and 49 • St 28–31 • Li 12 • Sp 13	Hip • Sacral • Coccygeal
Knees	St 34, 35, and 41 • UB 54 • GB 34, 39, and 40 • Li 4 and 8 • Sp 9	Knee
Thighs	GB 29–31 • UB 49	Hip • Knee
Shoulders	Co 15 • Me 14 • SI 9	Shoulder • Neck • Thoracic
Ankles	Sp 5 • St 41 • GB 40 • UB 59–62 • Ki 3–8	Ankle
Feet	GB 35 and 40 • UB 28, 58, and 59 • Ki 2 and 3 • St 31 • Sp 11	Ankle • Toes
Toes		
Great Toes	Sp 1–3 • Li 1–3	Toes
Second Toes	Li 2–4 • St 43–45	Toes
Middle Toes	Li 4 • GB 41	Toes
Fourth Toes	GB 42–44	Toes
Little Toes	UB 64–67	Toes
Connective Tissue Disorders Related to Arthritis		
Gout	St 36 • GB 34 • Co 8 and 9 • Me 6 • Arthritis points for specific areas	Sympathy • Shenmen • Liver • Kidney • Pancreas • Stomach • Small Intestine

Lupus Erythematosis

Skin Lesions Systemic	Co 4 and 11 · St 36 · Me 6 · Sp 6 · Va 3 · GB 20 · Br 20 · Lu 3 and 7 · He 2 and 5 · St 40 · Sp 5 and 11 · Va 2	Shenmen · Sympathy · Heart · Lung · Kidney · Liver · Pancreas
Polymyositis	Arthritis points for afflicted areas	Shenmen · Sympathy · Lung · Liver · Kidney · Points for afflicted areas
Reiter's Syndrome	St 36 · UB 11 · GB 1 · Arthritis points for afflicted areas	Shenmen · Sympathy · Urethra · Eye · Eye I and II · Liver · Kidney · Points for afflicted areas
Sjögren's Syndrome	Co 20 · Lu 7 and 9 · Br 24 and 25 · St 12 and 14 · Ki 20 · GB 33 and 43 · Li 6 · Sp 3 · Points for arthritic joints	Shenmen · Lung · Pharynx · Internal Nose · Maxillary Sinus · Points for afflicted joints
Cervical Syndromes General	SI 3 · UB 10, 60 and 62 · GB 20 and 37	Neck · Sympathy · Shenmen
Torticollis	St 9–12 · Co 4, 16–18 · Me 14–16 · GB 20 and 21 · UB 10 and 11 · Br 12–14	Neck · Shoulder · Brain · Lung · Sympathy
Whiplash Residuals	Lu 7 · Co 11, 15, and 16 · SI 3 and 19 · GB 39 · UB 10, 60, and 62 · GB 20 and 39	Neck · Shoulder · Lung · Sympathy · Shenmen
Disc and Spinal Abnormalities		
Cervical	Co 4 · SI 12–15 · UB 10–12 · Br 12 · St 13, 14, and 36 · Sp 6	Neck · Shoulder · Shenmen · Sympathy
Thoracic	Co 4, 14–16 · SI 14 and 15 · GB 25 · UB 12–22, 36–47 · Br 4–11	Thoracic · Lumbar · Shenmen
Lumbar-Sacral	Co 4 · St 36 · Br 3–5 · UB 20–28, 31, 47, and 48 · GB 30	Lumbar · Sacral · Coccygeal · Shenmen

SPECIFIC POINTS FOR VARIOUS CONDITIONS (Continued)

Medical Conditions	Points on Major Meridians	Auricular Points
Tendinitis and Tenosynovitis		
Arms and Hands	Co 5 • Lu 7 • Va 7 • He 7 • Arthritis points for involved joints	Shoulder • Elbow • Fingers • Kidney • Sympathy
Hips	GB 30, 31, and 34 • UB 30, 31, 48, and 49 • St 28–31 • Li 12 • Sp 13	Hip • Liver • Kidney • Sympathy
Knees	GB 34 • St 33–37 • Sp 9 and 10 • Li 7 and 8 • UB 52–55 • Ki 10	Knee • Liver • Kidney • Sympathy
Ankles	UB 59–62 • GB 39 and 40 • St 41 • Li 4 • Ki 3–8	Ankle • Liver • Kidney • Toes • Sympathy
Tennis Elbow	Co 5 • Lu 7 • Va 7 • He 7 • GB 34 • Co 11 and 12	Elbow • Shenmen • Sympathy
Muscle Strains and Spasms		
Neck	SI 3 • UB 10, 60 and 62 • GB 20 and 37	Neck • Shoulder • Shenmen
Shoulder	Co 14–16 • SI 3, 11, 12, and 19 • GB 21	Shoulder • Neck • Shenmen
Thoracic and Lumbar	SI 14 and 15 • UB 12–24 • 37–47 • St 36 • Sp 6	Thoracic • Lumbar • Kidney • Stomach • Shenmen
Arms and Hands	Lu 9 and 10 • Va 8 • Co 3 and 4 • Me 2–4 • GB 21	Fingers • Shoulder • Elbow • Neck • Sympathy
Lower Extremities	GB 30–40 • UB 49–59 • St 31–42 • Sp 8 and 10 • Li 6 and 9 • Ki 7–10	Hip • Knee • Ankle • Toes • Lumbar • Shenmen • Sympathy
Bursitis		
Shoulder	Co 11, 15, and 16 • SI 19 • GB 39	Shoulder • Shenmen
Elbow	Co 11 • St 36 • GB 21	Elbow • Shenmen

Condition	Points	Areas
Ischial Tuberosity	GB 30 · UB 30, 33–35, 48–50	Hip · Lumbar · Sacral
Heel	UB 60–62 · Ki 3–6 · Li 4 · Sp 5 and 6 · St 36 and 41	Ankle · Toes · Sacral

Neurologic Disorders

Impaired Function Syndromes

Condition	Points	Areas
Organic Brain Syndromes	St 25 and 36 · He 7 · UB 15, 18, and 20 · Br 4, 14, and 20 · Ki 4 · Sx 2, 5, 14, and 23 · Sp 3, 6 and 15 · Me 6	Brain · Lungs · Liver · Kidney · Spleen · Heart · Gonads
Amnesia	St 36 · He 7 · UB 15 · Co 4 · Br 20	Same as OBS above
Aphasia	Co 4 · St 6 · Sx 14 and 23	Same as OBS above
Dementia	Co 4 · St 6 and 36 · He 7 · UB 15 · Br 14 and 20	Same as OBS above
Coma	Br 20 and 26 · Sx 4 and 8 · Va 3, 6, and 9 · UB 15, 17, and 54 · He 7 · Li 3 · GB 30, 31, and 39 · Co 1,	Brain · Forehead · Shenmen · Sympathy Spleen · Kidney · Rectum
Hypersomnia	Br 26 · Sx 4 and 8 · He 7 · UB 15 · Va 6 and 9 · Li 3	Brain · Forehead · Spleen · Stomach · Liver · Kidney · Shenmen
Seizures	GB 2, 13, 20 and 40 · Me 3 and 5 · Co 4 and 10 · Br 20 and 26 · SI 3 and 19 · Li 2 · UB 15, 18, and 62 · Sx 12 · Sp 6 · St 40	Brain · Liver · Kidney · Shenmen · Sympathy

Impaired Sensory Perception

Condition	Points	Areas
Anosmia	Co 4 and 20 · Br 14, 16, 23, and 26 · SI 2 · UB 13	Brain · Kidney · Eye · Internal Nose
Glaucoma and Cataracts Blindness	GB 4–6, and 14 · St 2 · UB 2 and 3 · Me 4 · Li 4 · Sx 24	Eye · Eye I and II · Liver · Kidney
Neurogenic	Lu 10 · Co 14 · SI 17 and 18 · Li 3 · Br 20 and 24	Eye · Eye I and II · Brain · Liver · Kidney
Deafness, Neurogenic	Co 4 · SI 19 · UB 23 · Me 3, 5, 17 and 22 · GB 11 and 12	Brain · Pharynx · Eye II · Inner Ear

SPECIFIC POINTS FOR VARIOUS CONDITIONS (Continued)

Medical Conditions	Points on Major Meridians	Auricular Points
Tinnitus	Co 4 and 5 • SI 4 and 5 • UB 23 • Ki 6 • Va 9 • Me 17 • GB 11 and 12	Brain • Liver • Kidney • Shenmen • Inner Ear
Dizziness	*Front:* Br 24 • GB 14 • Li 14 • He 2 • Lu 6 • GB 24 • Sp 12 • St 36, 40, 41, and 44. *Back:* UB 8 • GB 9 and 21 • Br 14, 17, and 19 • Me 11 • Co 14 • Ki 6 and 10	Brain • Inner Ear • Liver • Kidney
Meniere's Disease	Points for Deafness • Tinnitus • Dizziness	Points for Deafness • Tinnitus • Dizziness
Numbness	St 36 • Sp 4 • Ki 1 • Br 25	Brain • Liver • Kidney
Upper Extremity	Co 10, 11, and 15 • GB 21	Neck • Elbow • Fingers
Lower Extremity	UB 23, 31 and 34 • GB 30, 31, 34, 36, and 39 • Ki 3 • Br 14	Lumbar • Sacral • Hip • Knee • Ankle • Toes
Impaired Motor Function		
Diaphragm	UB 17 • Li 14 • Sx 15	Diaphragm • Thoracic • Lung
Abdominal Muscles	UB 20 and 21 • St 21 and 25	Thoracic • Abdomen • Diaphragm • Lung • Hip
Upper Extremities	Ex 17 • Co 4, 6, 10, 11, and 15 • Me 5	Shoulder • Elbow • Fingers • Neck
Lower Extremities	Ex 21 • GB 30, 31, and 34 • UB 23 and 40 • Li 8 • St 36, 37, and 41 • Ki 3 • Sp 6	Lumbar • Sacral • Hip • Knee • Ankle • Toes
Urethral and Rectal Sphincters	Sx 4 • UB 32 and 54	Lumbar • Sacral • Hip • Urethra • Rectum • Brain • Urinary Bladder • Genitalia • Colon
Amyotrophic L.S.	Co 3, 5, and 7 • Lu 2, 3, 6, and 10 • St 5, 10, and 11 • Sp 8–10 • SI 10, 12, and 15 • Me 4, 9, 11, and 14 • Li 16–18 • Sx 22–24	Pharynx • Larynx • Diaphragm • Elbow • Finger • Neck • Thoracic • Lumbar • Liver • Lung

Multiple Sclerosis	GB 20, 30, and 33 • UB 23, 54, and 60 • Sp 6 and 9 • Ki 3 • St 36 • Br 2	Eye • Brain • Neck • Lumbar • Thoracic • Lung
Bell's Palsy	SI 2, 4, 6, and 7 • Co 10, 11, 19, and 20 • St 18 and 36 • Br 16, 20, and 23 • UB 1 and 2 • GB 1, 3, 14, and 15 • Me 5, 15, 17, 22, and 23 • Sp 6 • Sx 12	Eye I and II • Maxillary Sinus • Brain • Liver • External Nose • Pharynx
Cerebral Palsy	Co 4, 10, 11, and 15 • St 36 • UB 23 • Ki 1 and 3 • GB 31, 34, and 39 • Br 14 • Points for specific symptoms	Brain • Lung • Liver • Neck • Thoracic • Lumbar • Sacral • Stomach • Colon
Paralysis and Paresis	Points listed for impaired function of specific areas	
Stroke Residuals	Points listed for specific symptoms	
Dyskinesia	Lu 5 • Co 4, 11, and 15 • St 23 • UB 60 • Br 20 and 24	Brain • Liver • Kidney
Parkinsonism	Lu 5 • Co 4, 11, and 15 • Sp 6 • St 33 • UB 60 • SI 8 • He 3 • Me 3 • Va 3 and 7 • Ki 3 • GB 30 and 40 • Li 3 • Br 20 and 24	Brain • Liver • Kidney • Neck • Thoracic
Tremors	St 4 and 6 • UB 1 and 2 • Me 21 and 23 • Sp 6 • SI 18 • Sx 24 • Br 26 • GB 2	Brain • Liver • Kidney • Neck • Thoracic
Ataxia	Prone: UB 8 • GB 9 and 21 • Br 14, 17, and 19 • Me 11 • SI 15 • Ki 6 and 10 • Supine: Sx 14 • GB 14 • Li 14 • He 2 • Lu 6 • Ki 26 • Sp 12 • St 36, 40, 41, and 44	Brain • Inner Ear • Liver • Lumbar • Sacral
Incontinence	Co 4 • St 36 • Sp 6 • UB 23 • Sx 2 and 4 • Br 4 and 27	Brain • Lumbar • Sacral • Rectum • Urethra • Urinary Bladder
Hyperactivity (MBD)	Lu 4 • Co 11 • St 36 and 40 • Sp 4 • Va 6 • He 5 • GB 21 • Sx 4 • UB 17, 18, and 20	Brain • Neck • Sympathy
Pain Syndromes	Co 4, 11, and 15 • St 36 • UB 23 and 54 • GB 30, 34, and 54 • Br 14 • Points for analgesia of each area and for treating cause of pain	Brain • Shenmen • Sympathy • Thoracic • Lumbar • Sacral • Neck • Points for area of pain

SPECIFIC POINTS FOR VARIOUS CONDITIONS (Continued)

Medical Conditions	Points on Major Meridians	Auricular Points
Neuralgia and Neuritis	Points for analgesia of each area and for treating cause of pain	Points for area of pain • Shenmen • Sympathy
Causalgia	Co 11 • Va 5 • Me 6 • St 25 and 29 • Sp 14 and 15	Shenmen • Sympathy • Neck • Thoracic • Lumbar • Sacral • Liver • Kidney
Intercostal Neuralgia	Co 11 • Va 5 • Me 6 • GB 38 and 43 • Li 2	Neck • Thoracic • Lumbar • Diaphragm • Lung
Sciatic Neuralgia	St 36 • UB 23, 25, 31, 49, 50, 54, and 60 • GB 34 and 39 • Br 25	Lumbar • Sacral • Shenmen • Sympathy
Trigeminal Neuralgia	Co 4, 11, 19, and 20 • St 4, 6, 7, 8, 40, and 44 • UB 2 and 62 • Br 26 • Me 17 and 21 • SI 17, 18, and 19 • GB 3, 14 and 20	Maxillary Sinus • Eye I and II • Upper and Lower Teeth • Forehead • Shenmen • Sympathy
Herpes Zoster	Co 4 and 11 • Sp 6 and 10 • UB 11–14, 21, and 22	Shenmen • Sympathy
Facial	GB 1 and 2 • SI 19 • St 1 • Me 23	Forehead • Eye I and II
Thoracic	UB 15–20 • GB 24 and 25 • St 20–25 • Sp 16 • Li 14 and 16 on opposite side	Thoracic • Lung • Kidney • Diaphragm
Headache	Lu 7 • Co 4 • St 8, 29, 30, 36, 40, and 43 • Sp 5, 6, 8, and 9 • UB 2, 7, 23, 25, and 62 • Ki 1 and 3 • Me 4, 6, 15, and 23 • GB 4, 5, 7, 20, and 40 • Li 1–3, and 8 • Sx 6 • Br 16, 19, 20, and 23	Brain • Forehead • Liver • Kidney • Lung • Stomach • Small Intestine • Colon
Emergency Pain Relief		
Abdomen	St 36 • Sp 6 • Li 3 • Br 4 • GB 38 and 34 • Me 6	Abdomen • Lung • Sympathy
Arms	Co 11, 12, and 15 • GB 14 • Me 5 • St 19	Neck • Elbow • Fingers
Neck	Co 4 • St 6 and 44 • Va 6 • GB 20 and 39 • SI 6	Neck • Shenmen • Sympathy

Chest and Thoracic Spine	Co 3 and 4 • Va 6 • Me 5 and 8 • GB 34 • UB 65	Shenmen • Lung • Diaphragm • Kidney • Spleen • Liver • Thoracic
Lumbar and Pelvic	UB 23 and 40 • SI 6 • Br 26 • SI 3 • St 36	Lumbar • Sacral • Coccygeal • Rectum • Lung • Uterus • Urethra • Hip • Gonads • Genitalia
Hips and Sacral	St 36 and 40 • UB 59 • GB 30, 36, and 39 • Sp 6 • Li 5	Hip • Sacral • Coccygeal • Rectum • Genitalia
Shoulder	St 38 • UB 57 • Co 11, 15, and 16 • SI 10 • GB 34 • Me 14	Neck • Shoulder • Shenmen • Sympathy
Throat	Co 4 • St 6 and 44 • Va 6	Pharynx • Larynx • Neck • Lung • Shenmen
Mouth	Co 4 • St 5–7, 44 • Me 21	Upper and Lower Teeth • Pharynx • Shenmen
Head	SI 18 • SI 3 • St 43 • GB 8 and 41 • UB 2	Brain • Neck • Forehead • Lung • Eye • Shenmen
Eyes	Co 4 • St 2 • GB 14 and 20 • Me 5	Eye II • Lung • Shenmen
Ears	Co 4 • Me 3 and 17 • Va 3 • GB 43	
Nose	Co 4 and 20 • St 2 • Br 24	Pharynx • Internal Nose • External Nose • Maxillary Sinus • Lung

Psychiatric and Emotional

Neuroses

Anxiety	Lu 4 • Co 11 • St 36 and 40 • Sp 4 • He 3, 5, and 7 • UB 15, 17–19, and 23 • Va 4 • GB 20 and 21 • Sx 4, 9, and 12	Lung • Brain • Sympathy
Depression	Lu 5, 7, and 10 • Co 15 • St 25 and 44 • Sp 6 • He 6 • SI 3 • UB 11, 13, 19, 20, 23, 38, and 60 • Ki 6 • Va 5, 6, and 8 • Me 6 • GB 20 • Li 2	Lung • Brain • Shenmen

Affective Disorders

For Stability	Br 12–14, 16, and 23 • Lu 7 and 9 • St 37 • Co 9 • Va 4 and 5 • He 7 • Li 1 • Sx 12 and 15	Brain • Liver • Kidney • Spleen
Hyperactive Phase	Sp 1 and 6 • Lu 5 and 11 • Sx 14 and 24 • St 6 and 36 • Br 16	Shenmen • Sympathy • Liver

SPECIFIC POINTS FOR VARIOUS CONDITIONS (Continued)

Medical Conditions	Points on Major Meridians	Auricular Points
Insomnia	Lu 9 • Co 4 and 11 • Sp 4 • He 7 • Ki 1 and 3	Shenmen • Sympathy • Lung • Liver
Depressive Phase	Points above for depression	
Anorexia	St 36 • UB 18 and 20 • Ki 4	Brain • Stomach • Liver • Shenmen
	St 36 • UB 18 and 20 • Ki 2 • Li 2–4, and 14 • Sx 12	Brain • Liver • Lung
Snoring	GB 2, 20, and 40 • Br 26 • UB 15 and 18 • SI 19 • Sx 12	Brain • Sympathy • Pharynx • Internal Nose • Lung • Maxillary Sinus • Tonsil
Nervousness	Points for Anxiety	Points for Anxiety
Speech Disorders	Co 4 and 11 • St 6 and 36 • Sp 4 • Va 6 • GB 21 • Sx 6, 14 and 23 • Br 14 and 20	Pharynx • Larynx • Neck • Maxillary Sinus • Upper and Lower Teeth • Shenmen • Sympathy
Addictive Disorders		
Drug Dependence	St 8, 15, 25, and 40 • Sx 10, 12, 13, and 14 • Br 20 • GB 20 and 34 • Ki 1 • Sp 1 and 6 • Va 7 • Lu 7 • SI 3 • Me 6	Brain • Shenmen • Sympathy • Lung • Liver • Kidney • Spleen • Stomach
Alcoholism	Lu 7 • Co 4, 10, 11, and 15 • St 8, 25, 40, and 44 • Sp 1 and 6 • UB 10, 11, 15, 54, and 60 • Ki 1 • SI 3 • Me 6 • GB 20 and 34 • He 7 • Sx 4 • Br 20	Brain • Liver • Kidney • Spleen • Stomach
Smoking Addiction	Lu 4 and 7 • Co 4 and 13 • St 36 and 40 • Sp 8 • Br 24 • He 7 • Va 6	Shenmen • Lung • Abdomen • Pharynx • Kidney • Internal Nose • Kidney • Maxillary Sinus
Obesity	St 25 and 36 • Sp 6 and 9 • Me 6 • Sx 4, 6, 8, and 11 • Va 6 and 9	Lung • Liver • Kidney • Brain • Small Intestine • Colon
Autism	Lu 9 • Co 4 and 11 • Sp 6 and 10 • UB 1, 12, and 54 • GB 20 • Ki 6 • Va 5, 7, and 9 • Me 5 and 17 • Sx 23	Brain • Liver • Kidney • Stomach • Sympathy
Schizophrenia	Lu 9 • Co 4 and 11 • St 36 and 40 • Sp 6 and 10 • UB 1 • GB 2 and 20 • Ki 6 • Va 5 and 7 • Me 5 and 17 • Sx 23 • SI 19	Brain • Liver • Kidney • Stomach • Sympathy

ACUPUNCTURE EXAMINATION

For each of the following questions, one answer only is correct. Please indicate the correct answer by putting a, b, or c after the number of the question.

1. Which of the following should not be treated with acupuncture in the United States?

    a. Osteoarthritis of the cervical spine
    b. Cancer of the breast
    c. Obesity

2. Where is the acupuncture point known as *Hoku*, Colon 4, or Large Intestine 4 located?

    a. On the foot
    b. On the back
    c. On the hand

3.   Which is the best way to sterilize acupuncture needles?

    a.   Boiling in water
    b.   Soaking in alcohol
    c.   Autoclaving

4.   Where are most of the points of the lung meridian located?

    a.   On the upper extremities
    b.   On the chest
    c.   On the neck

5.   Where is acupuncture point Stomach 36, C 36, *Tsusanli* located?

    a.   On the abdomen
    b.   Near the elbow
    c.   Near the knee

6.   Where is point Stomach 31, C 31, *Pikuan* located?

    a.   At the base of the big toe
    b.   Just below the navel
    c.   On the thigh

7.   Which point is used most frequently for dental anesthesia?

    a.   Colon 4, Large Intestine 4, *Hoku*
    b.   Metabolism 7, Triple Warmer 7, J 7, *Tienching*
    c.   Liver 8, L 8, *Chuchuan*

8.   Which is a forbidden point for acupuncture?

    a.   Lung 11, A 11, *Shaoshang*
    b.   Stomach 36, C 36, *Tsusanli*
    c.   Brain 17, Governor Vessel 17, N 17, *Naohu*

9.   Which one of the following is not a forbidden point for acupuncture?

    a.   Stomach 17, C 17, *Juchung*
    b.   Gall Bladder 18, K 18, *Chengling*
    c.   Colon 1, Large Intestine 1, B 1, *Shanyang*

10.   Where is Spleen 4, D4, *Kungsun* located?

    a.   On the abdomen
    b.   On the foot
    c.   On the hand

11. Which of the following points is used to initiate labor in pregnancy?

    a. Colon 4, Large Intestine 4, *Hoku*

    b. Sex 23, Conception Vessel 23, M 23, *Lienchuan*

    c. Brain 16, Governor Vessel, N 16, *Fengfu*

12. Which meridian has the most acupuncture points?

    a. Urinary bladder, G, *Tsu Tai Yang Pang Kuang Ching*

    b. Lung, A, *Shou Tai Yin Fei Ching*

    c. Heart, E, *Shou Shao Yin Hsin Ching*

13. What should you do if a patient has a seizure?

    a. Give him hot tea

    b. Pour cold water on his face

    c. Notify a licensed physician

14. What should you do if a patient expresses lack of confidence in acupuncture?

    a. Give him the names and telephone numbers of patients you have treated in the past

    b. Listen to what he has to say and assure him you will try to do your best to help him

    c. Refuse to treat him

15. Which of the following blood pressures is normal?

    a. 120/80

    b. 180/120

    c. 80/50

16. Which of the following diseases may a patient get from improperly sterilized needles four months after acupuncture treatment?

    a. Hepatitis

    b. Typhoid fever

    c. Cellulitis

17. Which of the following should never be given to an unconscious patient?

    a. Hot tea by mouth

    b. Oxygen

    c. Acupuncture

18. Which of these drugs should not be discontinued while a patient has acupuncture treatments?

    a.   Insulin
    b.   Aspirin
    c.   Tylenol

19. What is the maximum amperage which is safe to use for electro-acupuncture?

    a.   Half ampere
    b.   Ten milliamperes
    c.   200 microamperes

20. How many moxibustion burns should be given for treating stomach pain?

    a.   Two or three
    b.   None
    c.   At least five

21. Which meridian has most points on the legs?

    a.   Urinary Bladder, G, *Tsu Tai Yang Pang Kuang Ching*
    b.   Colon, Large Intestine, B, *Shou Yang Min Ta Chang Ching*
    c.   Sex, Conception Vessel, M, *Jen Mo*

22. How deeply should acupuncture needles be inserted into the chest?

    a.   At least four centimeters
    b.   Usually about three centimeters
    c.   Less than one centimeter

23. Which of the following is likely to be relieved by acupuncture treatments?

    a.   Brain tumor
    b.   Varicose veins
    c.   Trigeminal neuralgia

24. To treat asthma, where should the needles be inserted?

    a.   Into the lungs
    b.   Into the liver
    c.   Not into any vital organ

25. Which of the following diseases should not be treated by acupuncture in the United States?

    a.   Migraine headaches

b.   Osteoarthritis
c.   Malaria

26. Which meridian has its first point on the sole of the foot?

a.   Kidney, H, Ki, *Tsu Shao Yin Sheng Ching*
b.   Brain, Governor Vessel, N, Br, *Tu Mo*
c.   Metabolism, Triple Warmer, J, Me, *Shou Shao Yang San Chiao Ching*

27. Which of the following meridians is not paired?

a.   Gall Bladder, K, GB, *Tsu Sho Yang Tan Ching*
b.   Spleen, D, Sp, *Tsu Tai Yin Pi Ching*
c.   Sex, Conception Vessel, M, Sx, *Jen Mo*

28. Which of the following meridians has points on the lateral aspect of the leg?

a.   Colon, Large Intestine, B, Co, *Shou Yang Min Ta Chang Ching*
b.   Spleen, D, Sp, *Tsu Tai Yin Pi Ching*
c.   Stomach, C, St, *Tsu Yang Ming Wei Ching*

29. Which of the following meridians has points on the lumbar area of the back?

a.   Sex, Conception Vessel, M, Sx, *Jen Mo*
b.   Brain, Governor Vessel, N, Br, *Tu Mo*
c.   Colon, Large Intestine, B, Co, *Shou Yang Min Ta Chang Ching*

30. Which of the following meridians does not have points on the arm?

a.   Heart, E, He, *Shou Shao Yin Hsin Ching*
b.   Sex, Conception Vessel, M, Sx, *Jen Mo*
c.   Lung, A, Lu, *Shou Tai Yin Fei Ching*

31. What is the generic name of the plant used for moxibustion?

a.   *Artemesia vulgaris*
b.   *Moxaba canubius*
c.   *Cannabis sativa*

32. Which of the following is not on the arm or hand?

a.   Heart 5, E 5, He 5, *Tungli*
b.   Lung 10, A 10, Lu 10, *Yuchi*
c.   Liver 2, L 2, Li 2, *Hsingchien*

33. What important structure should be avoided under acupuncture point Lung 7, A 7, *Liehchueh*?

   a. Radial artery
   b. Sciatic nerve
   c. The lung

34. What important structure should be avoided under acupuncture point Urinary Bladder 38, G 38, *Kaohuang?*

   a. Radial artery
   b. Urinary Bladder
   c. Lung

35. What important structure should be avoided near acupuncture point Gall Bladder 1, K 1, GB 1, *Tungtzuliao?*

   a. Mouth
   b. Eye
   c. Esophagus

36. What important structure should be avoided near point Metabolism 23, J 23, *Szuchukung?*

   a. Mouth
   b. Eye
   c. Urinary bladder

37. What important structure should be avoided under point Spleen 15, D 15, *Taheng?*

   a. Sciatic nerve
   b. Eye
   c. Intestine

38. What important structure should be avoided under Gall Bladder 14, K 14, *Yangpai?*

   a. Frontal air sinus
   b. Gall bladder
   c. Kidney

39. Which of the following acupuncture points is not usually used to treat obesity?

   a. Stomach 36, C 36, *Tsusanli*
   b. Vascular 6, Triple Warmer 6, I 6, *Neikuan*
   c. Colon 20, Large Intestine 20, B 20, *Yinghsiang*

40. Which of the following is not usually used in acupuncture for tinnitus?

a.   Colon 5, Large Intestine 5, B 5, *Yanghsi*
b.   Lung 11, A 11, *Shaoshang*
c.   Small Intestine 4, F 4, *Wanku*

41. What structure is located just above the kidney?

a.   Adrenal gland
b.   Thyroid gland
c.   Pituitary gland

42. Which of the following pulse rates would be considered normal?

a.   72
b.   50
c.   40

43. Which wave form should not be used for electro-acupuncture?

a.   Sine wave
b.   Sawtooth wave
c.   Square wave

44. For which condition is it advisable to penetrate the chest and enter the lung with acupuncture needles?

a.   Bronchial asthma
b.   None
c.   Emphysema

45. Why is it important to establish a diagnosis before giving acupuncture?

a.   Some more effective alternative treatment might be available.
b.   American patients like to know the name of their disease.
c.   It is not important.

46. What information can an electro-acupuncture instrument give?

a.   Identification of the meridian
b.   The skin resistance
c.   The diagnosis of the patient's disease

47. Where is acupuncture point Small Intestine 6, F 6, *Yanglao* located?

a.   On the abdomen
b.   On the arm
c.   On the leg

48. Where is acupuncture point Urinary Bladder 51, G 51, *Yenmen* located?
    a. On the lower part of the abdomen, near the midline
    b. On the middle part of the back
    c. On the back of the thigh

49. Where is acupuncture point Metabolism 2, Triple Warmer 2, J 2, *Yemen* located?
    a. On the back of the hand
    b. Near the mouth
    c. On the abdomen, upper quadrants

50. For which diseases can an acupuncturist guarantee a cure?
    a. Nerve deafness
    b. Rheumatoid arthritis
    c. None

True and False

1. Cleansing and soaking needles in alcohol is the best way to sterilize them.

2. If a patient loses consciousness during treatment, he should be given some hot tea to drink.

3. The *Hoku* or Colon 4 points are usually used for dental anesthesia.

4. Burning a patient with moxibustion can cause serious medical problems.

5. Patients receiving acupuncture should discontinue all the drugs they are taking.

6. A large artery is located near the surface of the skin just in front of the ear.

7. Sometimes it is helpful to puncture the eardrum to treat nerve deafness.

8. Most of the points of the lung meridian are located on the front of the chest wall.

9. The colon or large intestine meridian begins on the index finger and terminates near the nose.

10. Most of the acupuncture points on the heart meridian are located on the arm.

11. The most frequently used points on the small intestine meridian are located on the abdomen.

12. The fifth point of the urinary bladder meridian is located on the head.

13. Some points on the kidney meridian are located on the abdomen.

14. No points of the kidney meridian are located on the feet.

15. The first point of the vascular (pericardium or heart governor) meridian is located on the middle finger.

16. The first point of the metabolism (triple warmer) meridian is located on the fourth finger.

17. More than 18 points of the gall bladder meridian are on the head.

18. The liver meridian has its first point on the great toe.

19. The sex (conception vessel) meridian and the stomach meridian are both paired.

20. The gall bladder meridian has more acupuncture points than the liver meridian.

21. The liver is like wood, and, therefore, does not have a large blood supply.

22. Acupuncture points in the outer ear are only useful for treating nerve deafness or for weight reduction.

23. Most of the major meridians are paired.

24. Acupuncture points are located in positions to facilitate piercing major nerves.

25. Acupuncture should not be used to treat mental illness in the United States.

26. Acupuncture should not be used to treat bacterial infections in the United States.

27. If a patient gets an infection from an acupuncture needle, it will be apparent within three days.

28. Hepatitis infections from needles may not make a patient sick until three months after the needles were inserted into his body.

29. Autoclaving and dry heat sterilizing are the best ways to sterilize acupuncture needles.

30. A good way to clean skin at the points of insertion of an acupuncture needle is by using alcohol-soaked cotton.

31. Inserting needles four centimeters into certain acupuncture points on the chest is good treatment for bronchial asthma.

32. It is important to avoid inserting acupuncture needles into arteries.

33. When patients are being treated with cortisone, they are likely to get hematomas from acupuncture.

34. Patients should be advised to stop taking cortisone when they begin acupuncture treatment.

35. Pulse diagnosis is adequate for ruling out the possibility of cancer.

36. A person who has had the same type of migraine headaches for 20 years is unlikely to have a brain tumor.

37. It may be a good prognostic sign if a patient has increased pain after his first acupuncture treatment.

38. Acupuncture can relieve leg paralysis if the patient gets enough treatments even if his spinal cord has been severed.

39. Acupuncture can relieve the pain and stiffness of osteoarthritis.

40. Acupuncture should not be used to treat parasitic infestations in the United States.

41. Acupuncture should not be used to treat cerebral palsy.

42. Gold acupuncture needles are more effective than those made of stainless steel.

43. Whether to use gold, silver, or stainless steel acupuncture needles should be determined by the disease for which treatment is to be given.

44. Burning patients with moxibustion is not an acceptable practice in the United States.

45. Most useful acupuncture points are located at least three centimeters under the skin.

46. The Large Intestine meridian is paired with the Small Intestine meridian.

47. Patients get better results from acupuncture if the acupuncturist guarantees a cure.

48. If a patient has swollen ankles, acupuncture needles should be inserted into his ankles to let the water come out after the needles are withdrawn.

49. Some of the points of the brain (governor vessel) meridian are located on the arms.

50. Some of the points of the gall bladder meridian are located on the head.

ANSWERS FOR ACUPUNCTURE EXAMINATION

Multiple Choice				*True and False*		
1. b	18. a	35. b		1. false	18. true	35. false
2. c	19. c	36. b		2. false	19. false	36. true
3. c	20. b	37. c		3. true	20. true	37. true
4. a	21. a	38. a		4. true	21. false	38. false
5. c	22. c	39. c		5. false	22. false	39. true
6. c	23. c	40. b		6. true	23. true	40. true
7. a	24. c	41. a		7. false	24. false	41. false
8. c	25. c	42. a		8. false	25. false	42. false
9. c	26. a	43. a		9. true	26. true	43. false
10. b	27. c	44. b		10. true	27. false	44. true
11. a	28. c	45. a		11. false	28. true	45. false
12. a	29. b	46. b		12. true	29. true	46. false
13. c	30. b	47. b		13. true	30. true	47. false
14. b	31. a	48. c		14. false	31. false	48. false
15. a	32. c	49. a		15. false	32. true	49. false
16. a	33. a	50. c		16. true	33. true	50. true
17. a	34. c			17. true	34. false	

INDEX

E

F

G

H